Nature's Superfood

The Blue-Green Algae Revolution

DEDICATION
To my parents, Allan and Elsie Corkindale

ACKNOWLEDGEMENTS
There are many people who helped me with this book. Many distributors of blue-green algae generously gave their time to explain its mysteries: thanks to Bernadette Griffin, David Howell and Sonia VanderDol of AquaSource; Ian Perkins of Nature's Gold; Mark Tracey of Hunter Ridgeley and Neil Dickson of All Seasons Healthcare. Bob MacElroy of NASA was a fund of information. I am also indebted to the people who wrote with their experiences of blue-green algae. Their stories are included in Chapter Nine.

I would like to give my wholehearted thanks to my agent, Serafina Clarke, for her enthusiasm and belief in the project and to Michael Alcock and Gordon Wise at Boxtree Macmillan, who were always fun, friendly – and frighteningly efficient. Liz Fergusson cleared up some of the aberrations in the manuscript and Rita Winter gave it a final polish.

Finally, thanks to my brother, Neil, and sister, Janet, for their help. Last, but not least, a big thank-you to Simon Freeman, who held out a much-needed hand of friendship through my darkest days.

Nature's Superfood

The Blue-Green Algae Revolution

GILLIAN CRIBBS

NEWLEAF

First published 1997 by Newleaf
an imprint of Macmillan Publishers Ltd
25 Eccleston Place, London SW1W 9NF
and Basingstoke

Associated companies throughout the world

ISBN 0 7522 0569 2

1 3 5 7 9 8 6 4 2

A CIP catalogue entry for this book is available from the
British Library

Typeset by SX Composing DTP, Rayleigh, Essex
Printed and bound in Great Britain by
Mackays of Chatham plc, Chatham, Kent

CONTENTS

PROLOGUE

A personal tribute to blue-green algae

> *Our health is as a voyage and every illness is an adventure story.*
>
> Margiad Evans, *A Ray of Darkness* (1952)

There are many good reasons for getting to know blue-green algae, as this book will show. As the oldest living organism on the planet – and one which could survive even a nuclear holocaust – it can teach us a few things about living. For millennia, it has been valued as a highly nutritious food source and today, on the eve of the twenty-first century, it is at the cutting edge of research into treatment for the biggest killers of the century – heart disease, cancer and AIDS.

Although my main purpose in writing this book is to explain how this remarkable organism can help people maintain and recover their most precious asset – health – I also have another, more personal, reason for writing this book. Until my late twenties, illness was not a word that had ever entered my vocabulary. I come from a robust, healthy family who had never experienced any serious illness. In fact, like many people, we considered illness to be something of a failure, particularly stress and nervous disorders.

However, out of the blue (or so I thought), at twenty-eight years old, I found myself in the grip of a debilitating, stress-related illness, which my friends and family could not understand and which doctors finally admitted they could not treat. The illness had a devastating effect on my life – I lost my career, my marriage, my home, my friends and, for a time, my sanity.

Despite all the chaos it wreaked in my life, I unexpectedly found myself on a journey of self-discovery which continues today. As well as making me more aware of health issues, the experience has forged a certain humility and compassion in me which I never possessed before. The trigger for this remarkable change in my life, which led me out of the shadows of illness into vibrant, glowing health, was blue-green algae.

I hope my story will inspire you to do everything you can do to maintain your health if you are well and to follow your own journey back to natural health if you are ill.

Journey to health

The onset of my illness began one ordinary morning in March 1989, when I awoke early, overcome with a half-understood notion that something had irrevocably changed. Lying in the warmth of my bed, I sleepily tried to flex my arms and legs, but felt a strange torpor and heaviness. I tried a few times, but it was no better.

I strained to lift my arms above the duvet and noticed that my hands seemed to be locked in a claw-like grip. Panic began to well up in me. There was a strange dank smell in the room and as I tried to sit up, I felt a numbness and heaviness in my legs and back. I could not even hold my head up. I lay back on the pillow, frightened and exhausted.

Through a cloud of pain, the memory of the previous night suddenly crystallized in my mind. Sharp jolts of an unfamiliar pain had woken me from sleep, searing through my arms and legs. My back had convulsed in spasms and I had felt a violent pain, like lightning bolts, shooting through my body and down my spine. The pain grew to the point where I almost passed out. Soon, I was only aware of myself floating above my body and observing myself convulsing in pain on the bed.

After ten minutes or so, the pain started to recede and I noticed that my body was pouring with an unpleasant-smelling sweat. I tried to get out of bed, but I did not have the strength. Exhausted, I fell into a deep and disturbing sleep.

That morning, it took three hours to get out of bed. Each time I tried to get up, the effort drained me and triggered the horrific, shooting pain in my back. Eventually, I managed to get dressed and struggled to the doctor's surgery. A walk that would have taken five minutes when I had been well, took me more than an hour that day.

My doctor was puzzled when she saw me; although it was obvious that I was in some distress, she seemed unsure of the diagnosis. In the end, having examined my arms, she signed me off work for three weeks, diagnosing tenosynovitis (inflammation of the tendons in my arms and wrists). The muscle spasm in my arms and upper body stress was so severe that it had affected my legs and back.

During the next few days, I watched in despair as my symptoms worsened: I could not walk, I had to rest most of the day and I was unable to even brush my teeth or lift a spoon or tea cup. I soon realized with horror that I was crippled. I could not use my hands or arms and found it an effort to walk. Alarmed, I arranged to see a consultant, who diagnosed repetitive strain injury (RSI), the umbrella term for complaints including tennis elbow, tenosynovitis, muscle strain and back problems. In my case, I suffered almost complete paralysis in the arms, lower back pain, and neck strain that left me unable to hold my head erect.

I was ordered to rest for six months and attend physiotherapy five times a week. The only reason I could come up with for the illness was the extreme pressure I had been under at work, where I had worked for long hours at a computer keyboard without an ergonomically designed chair or desk. My consultant believed that the hours I had spent straining to see the screen and use the keyboard had forced me into an unnatural posture which my body had eventually been unable to sustain. Unfortunately, RSI is not recognized in the UK and I had to fight hard to persuade my company to allow me to have time off for treatment.

I underwent months of physiotherapy, which had little effect. My limp arms were covered with bundles of towels filled with ice cubes until they 'burned' with the cold. After six months, I had intensive ultrasound and massage and when this proved ineffective, I was told that there was no other treatment, save electric shock treatment or steroid injections in my fingertips. I decided if these were the only options available to me, it was time to find my own way through this terrible illness.

During those early months, I inevitably spent many hours alone. Life became increasingly difficult for me as I lost all memory of what it was like to live a normal life – to do simple, everyday things, like washing my hair, going to work, writing a letter, driving a car or even cooking a meal. As a student, I had prided myself on being able to take verbatim longhand notes at lectures; now I couldn't even sign a cheque.

At work, I had thought nothing of sitting at a keyboard typing for ten hours at a stretch; now I couldn't sit for more than ten minutes. Nor could I bear anyone shaking my hand or even coming near me in case they accidentally knocked my tender arms. Standing in a crowded tube train, jostling with people was something that filled me with dread.

I found this sudden helplessness quite terrifying and incomprehensible. Not surprisingly, I soon became depressed and anxious, something which I found more and more difficult to hide from friends and family who visited me. In the early days of my illness, they had shown great sympathy, but I noticed that after a few months, they had either lost interest or had grown irritated with me. Soon, even my closest friends and relations accused me of malingering and making up my symptoms.

One of the problems with stress-related illnesses, like RSI or ME, is that the only thing you can do to try and recover is to rest. But this tends to reinforce the idea that people who suffer from these illnesses are malingerers who are imagining their symptoms – the more relaxed I looked, the harder people found it to believe I was ill.

After a while, my visitors dwindled and offers of help faded away. My family, too, became exasperated with me; one day my mother asked, in complete frustration, just how long this illness was going to go on. I did not have the heart to tell her that it might very well go on for the rest of my life.

During those months of growing isolation, I began to torture myself psychologically. At first, I was angry and frustrated that this had happened to me. Why me? I kept asking myself. As I spent endless, solitary days at home, I began to lose my sense of place or time. All I could do was rack my brain for a reason why it had happened. On my darkest days, I sank into a deep, engulfing depression which only sleep could heal. On better days, I tried to think back to the time when I had felt really healthy and began to chart in my mind my descent from health into illness.

After a few months, when my anger had subsided, I began to look back over the last few years for signs of an incipient illness. Soon, a pattern began to emerge in my mind. The warning signs had been there all along, but I had been so out of touch with my body – as many people are – that I had never acknowledged the onset of illnesses or pieced together the symptoms that were clues to a gradual decline.

I had brushed aside any bouts of illness with a disdain I now find incredible; I simply assumed that they were meaningless and that I would return to the perfect health that was my birthright. Of course, I was very wrong.

Remembering my healthy years was easy; one day immediately came to mind – New Year's Eve, 1986. I had touched down at a wet and windy Heathrow airport from Cyprus, where I had spent two sunshine-filled years. My husband and I had had an exciting time there; he was a British diplomat and I had worked for the *Middle East Times* and later a local publisher, for whom I had written a travel guide to the island.

We had had a healthy outdoor life, passing endless sunny days swimming in the sparkling Mediterranean or picnicking in the Troodos and Kyrenia Mountains. Food was fresh, plentiful and cheap and the air was pure and clean. When we returned home that night in December 1986, we were both brimming with life and vitality.

Two months later, after a cold and miserable English winter, I was feeling less than sunny. I was working long and stressful hours as a journalist and, before long, my life revolved around four things: sleep; commuting; work; and weekday visits to the wine bar. My husband worked even longer hours at the Foreign Office, so we rarely dined together; we snatched meals at odd times and ate more and more convenience food. On many evenings, after a few glasses of wine, I didn't bother to eat at all.

The following year, I changed jobs and worked even longer hours, travelling twice as far to the office. To relieve the stress, I went out for drinks nearly every evening and snatched food as and when I could. Anyone who lives or works in a city, particularly London, would recognize this lifestyle. It was fast, fun, slightly irresponsible — exactly the pattern most young adults in their early careers fall into. Many twentysomethings get away with it. Others, like myself, are not so lucky.

By December 1988, exactly two years after I had returned to London, I realized that I had begun to feel tired and unwell. Throughout that month, I had struggled through the day, only to fall into bed exhausted when I got home. The office Christmas party that year stood out in my mind; I remembered feeling strangely detached from the group of people I was talking to. I felt cold and tired and suddenly could not bear the noise of the party. I went straight home to bed.

That night, my entire body ached and I broke out in a feverish sweat. When I awoke the next day, I felt a torpor in my limbs. I could not bear the light from the window and my appetite had all but vanished. I remember staying in bed for the rest of the holiday, unable to eat or drink anything.

As my mind raced over these events, I began to wonder whether this was, indeed, the onset of my illness. I vaguely recalled returning to work without having fully recovered. As many people do, I forced myself to get up in the morning, drive to work (I could no longer stand the noise of trains screeching to a halt at stations) and struggle through the day in a mental fog. I would skip lunch and dinner because I still had no appetite and by eight o'clock I was completely exhausted. I would then sleep a full twelve hours through to the next morning, only feeling just as shattered when I awoke, barely able to drag myself out of bed and begin the whole daily cycle again.

My doctor's advice was to give up work and take vitamin C supplements. She said, unhelpfully, that she thought I was a hypochondriac (I had once told her that I worked for a medical journal). It was clear even then that she had no idea – and even less patience – about what was wrong with me. It was not something I could discuss with my husband or family, who all enjoyed good health and had no real understanding of illness. In desperation, I decided to take a holiday in the hope that it would give me the boost I needed. I took three weeks off and flew to Canada, where my sister lived.

Looking back at the photographs I have of myself during that holiday, I find it incredible that none of the people around me ever mentioned how ill I looked. I had a husband, friends, colleagues, family, but no one listened to me or believed me when I said I was feeling unwell. I had always been strong and healthy; in the space of a few months, it seemed, I had become an empty, lifeless shell. My hair had fallen out in handfuls. I had lost a stone at least in weight, my skin was grey and my eyes were sunken. I could not bear extremes of noise, temperature or light. For most of the trip around Canada, I slept and ate, to my sister's despair. But, when I collapsed with exhaustion at Montreal airport, she realized that something was seriously wrong.

When I returned to the UK, my doctor again advised me to change my lifestyle and take more vitamins. I carried on working until early the following year, by which time I was experiencing constant pain in my neck, arms and back and a strange sense of an incipient paralysis creeping down my left side. When I visited my doctor, worried that I might have experienced a minor stroke, she laughed and said I was simply working too hard.

Perhaps she was right: the magazine had introduced computers the previous autumn and we had all been under great pressure at work to produce the magazine on a badly programmed system. She authorized X-rays and endless blood tests, but could find nothing wrong. She clearly thought my complaint was psychosomatic and implied that I was wasting valuable consultation time when she had seriously ill patients to attend to.

In many ways, the world conspires against patients like me. I was young, happily married and had a good career. The question everybody was asking, was what on earth did I have to worry about? Many people had far more serious problems than I did. It was true, I had to agree. So I ignored the symptoms – but with disastrous consequences.

At the end of six months' physiotherapy, I resigned from my job and started to do occasional days on various newspapers. By that time, I was suffering the secondary effects of RSI; as my muscles began to relax, my circulation was left impaired and the damage to my ner... ...had a knock-on effect on my digestive system, leaving r... ...estive disorders and irritable bowel syndrome, w... ...of careful treatment to manage. Howev... ...back and arms eased off, I took... advice of my physiotherapi... each day and was the onl... under control.

I also tried man... shiatsu, aromathera... spiritual healing... therapy seemed t... for more than... progress disar...

Soon, I...

to have expensive treatment after every day I worked, which eventually became uneconomical. All I could do was continue with yoga, eat a low-fat, vegetarian diet and take up meditation to preserve my sanity.

The combination of unemployment, a solitary existence and an illness doctors tell you they cannot treat – or else deny exists – is a dangerous one. I spiralled further into depression and began to lose all sense of reality. Increasingly, I began to rely on meditation as this alone provided an escape from my desperate situation. I also focused on my diet, believing that this was the only sure way back to health. I had only these two hopes to cling to as my life was cut further and further adrift.

In the end, yoga was both my salvation and downfall. Although the exercises ironed out my crumpled limbs and improved my state of mind, it also left me highly strung and rather sensitive. I also followed an exclusively vegetarian diet and before long I could not tolerate food that was not completely natural (as we shall see later, very little modern food is 100 per cent pure). Eventually, it became such an obsession that I could not even bear to be among people who did not share my vision of health.

After a while, my enforced pure lifestyle meant that I found it hard to function in the real world; every time I walked outdoors, I was assailed by traffic fumes and pollution, which I could actually taste as I breathed in the air.

The lack of adequate protein – especially animal protein – meant I was extremely light-headed. One yoga teacher, the problem, warned me to increase my protein that without protein to ground us, we can fly ons, floating above reality and in danger the world. He told me to eat anyng myself back down to earth.

I took his advice and, not surprisingly, all the old symptoms returned. But I did not mind; I made a decision that it was better to live in the real world and cope with my illness than to withdraw from the world and try to create an ivory tower for myself. I also decided that, RSI or not, it was time to get my career back on track. I practised handwriting for a few weeks and, working through the pain, managed eventually to write a few sentences. I picked up my tape recorder and notebook and went out to look for stories. This moment, I realized later, was the turning point in my life – I was about to discover blue-green algae for myself.

It was the summer of 1991. My first assignment was to interview an American management 'guru' at the Royal Masonic Hospital in west London, who was running a weekend workshop on how to develop one's intuition. He was a psychic who had a reputation in the US for helping managers of blue-chip companies use their intuition to make business decisions. It seemed like a good story and I went to listen to his lecture on the Sunday morning.

At 11am we broke for coffee and as I wandered over to a group of people standing in the shade of a huge oak tree – it was a blisteringly hot day – I felt a light tap on my shoulder. I turned to find an elderly woman, small and slim, with long grey hair and sharp blue eyes.

She told me her name was Claire and that she had something to tell me. Intrigued, I walked with her away from the main group and we sat underneath another oak tree. She told me she was clairvoyant and was about to go into a trance. 'I am being told that you have a problem with your health,' she began. 'Your arms. I don't understand what this means,' she continued, 'but I am getting the words blue-green algae. Do you understand what I am saying?' She opened her eyes and stared at me intently. 'Was that helpful?' she asked.

I had to confess, I had not understood what she said. I had never heard of blue-green algae and had a funny vision of myself swimming among whales in the deep ocean, scooping up vast mouthfuls of plankton.

She laughed too when she saw me smiling, although she later told me she hadn't known why, as she never remembered what she told people in trance. When I told her she had said I needed blue-green algae, she confessed to never having heard of it either. 'Could it be a health food?' she asked later, in another moment of inspiration.

I never met Claire again, but over the next few months, I tried hard to find out about blue-green algae. I went into every health-food shop I could find in London, but each time I asked for it, I was met with a blank stare of incomprehension. No one had even heard of it. After months and months of fruitless enquiries, I gave up.

As the years rolled on, I managed to stabilize my condition: some yoga, swimming, a good diet. I was able to do a few days' work each month and slowly I began to carve out a life that approximated to my old life. By that time, I had divorced. My husband had not been able to come to terms with my illness. I think he secretly regarded me as a depressed, introverted malingerer and simply waited for this 'phase' to pass. His perception of me was, sadly, shared by many others, including close friends and family. My circle of friends had shrunk dramatically, as fewer and fewer were prepared to accept me in my new state. My life had become pitifully proscribed for a thirty-year-old woman, but I was thankful that I had, at least, escaped those terrible days spent staring at the wall in despair.

Three years of this existence passed until the summer of 1995 when, quite unexpectedly, I had a breakthrough. I had arranged to meet a friend at the Hale Clinic, an alternative health clinic in central London. I arrived ten minutes early and decided to browse around the bookshop in the basement. The books were at the back of the health-food store and, as I walked through, a sign on one of the lower shelves caught my eye. I knelt down to have a closer look and spotted a wedge of leaflets on blue-green algae.

I felt my heart beat with anticipation as I read the leaflet. It said blue'green algae was the oldest – and purest – food on earth. It was related to plankton, which supported, among other sea creatures, the great blue whale. Suddenly, my vision of swimming with whales made sense. I cast my eye over the impressive list of vitamins, minerals and amino acids – I had never seen so many nutrients in a single food. And, although I balked at the price a little (£17 for a small jar), I decided to buy some.

The rest, as they say, is history. I believe that in all our lives there are defining moments, when we do something – good or bad – that will affect us for years to come. Buying blue-green algae that day at the Hale Clinic was a defining moment for me. Although I cannot honestly claim to have enjoyed its taste, I persevered and am eternally grateful that I did.

I was still suffering chronic symptoms of RSI – tense, locked muscles, fatigue, poor circulation and low appetite. I had long ago accepted that my health and strength would never be more than 65–70 per cent of what it had been. However, the first time I took blue-green algae, I felt a subtle change occur within myself. It is hard to define precisely where this happened – in my mind or body – all I can say is that I experienced a powerful 'shift' within myself. It was as though the physical and mental parts of myself – which had always operated independently – had merged into one. Suddenly, I felt more powerful and strong, as if the two parts had somehow reinforced each other. From that position of strength, there followed a gradual clearing of my mind.

After a week, an unexpected frisson of energy returned to my body, for the first time in nine years. It was a subtle, tingling flow, as if my blood had been supercharged and was flowing freely — not sluggishly as was usual — around my body. I had an instinct that it was the return of the subtle life force, which yogis describe as 'prana' and the Chinese call 'Chi'.

After a month, I noticed a considerable improvement in my mental clarity and a great surge in energy levels. Low reserves of energy had been one of the most worrying things about my illness, and the thing which had been the most difficult to manage. There had been times during my illness when I had been unable even to walk to the end of the road as I had so little energy. Worse, it had been a terrifying realization that I had no reserves of energy left — I felt like there was a battery powering me that had completely lost its life and could not be recharged. This was the real miracle of blue-green algae for me — it restored that reserve of energy and took away the fear of doing things, ultimately handing back control of my life to me.

As the months progressed, the chronic health problems that I had resigned myself to coping with for the rest of my life slowly — and miraculously — began to fade away. The tension in my neck and back, which had left my shoulders and upper back completely rigid, began to ease. This was the biggest surprise of all, as I had spent endless (expensive!) hours at the physiotherapist, having deep tissue massage, which had only brought relief for an hour or so after the treatment. My circulation began to improve too; for the first time in eight years, my feet and hands felt warm to the touch and I no longer had to pile on layers of clothes to keep warm.

As the chronic conditions began to improve, I noticed several other beneficial effects. My skin was clearer than it had been for years, my hair became glossy again and my eyes sparkled. Most interesting of all, however, was the fact that my craving for sweets and chocolates seemed to disappear overnight – and with it the excess weight (and cellulite) I had been trying to shift for years.

As well as these important physical changes, I also began to feel a greater sense of self-awareness. At first, this took the form of powerful dreams and painful buried feelings rising up from my subconscious, forcing me to confront them. Once this stage had passed, however, a sense of calm descended on me and I began to feel steadier than I had done for a long time. I returned to meditation feeling more grounded than I did years before.

Today I feel better than I have done for years. I have a full-time job, write books and articles in my spare time, socialize as much as possible with friends and exercise most days. I still take blue-green algae once or twice a day to maintain my health and mental well-being. As you can see, it has turned my life around completely – I hope that you, too, will benefit from improved health and stamina when you embark on your own journey back to health.

INTRODUCTION

The blue-green algae revolution

*Yesterday is but a dream, tomorrow is but a vision. But
today well lived makes every yesterday a dream of happiness
and every tomorrow a dream of hope.*

Sanskrit proverb

Thirty years ago, the race to send the first man to the moon
had a dramatic and defining effect on popular culture in the
West. Space-age fashions were in vogue and a whole new
genre of films, books and songs emerged, as the world's imag-
ination was seized by the seemingly infinite opportunities that
space travel presented.

For the first time, people caught a glimpse of the twenty-
first century, when in their fantasies, they could all fly to the
moon, travel beyond our solar system and exist on a handful
of supervitamins.

Now, as we stand on the threshold of the twenty-first
century and a new millennium, we are no closer to holidays
on the moon, but somehow, the idea of discovering a super-
food that would meet all our nutritional needs has remained
a tantalizing possibility. Of course, few people would like to
exchange one of life's greatest pleasures for a handful of pills,
yet the idea of finding a food that would give us quick, complete nutrition retains a certain appeal as our lives become
ever more stressful.

Scientists and nutritionists also dream of discovering a substance which would help us to become fit and healthy without having to understand the complexities of eating a well-balanced diet. If that substance could also boost our energy levels, give vegetarians and athletes the extra nutrients they require and help slimmers lose weight, it would completely change the way the food industry operates.

If such a substance could also act as a preventive supplement against degenerative and incurable diseases and conditions, such as cancer, multiple sclerosis, chronic fatigue syndrome, heart disease and osteoporosis, it would provoke nothing short of a revolution in medicine. And if it could be grown cheaply, without using too many precious natural resources, it could provide the answer to the world food crisis.

In the West, over-refined food, chemical residues and pollution are leaving us severely malnourished and in poor health. People are desperate to find a way through the maze of contradictory information about food and health supplements. Food in our shops is less nutritious than even twenty years ago and hard-edged marketing campaigns brainwash us into believing that the only way to maintain our health is to buy expensive vitamin supplements. Health is no longer everyone's birthright – it has become a multimillion pound industry feeding on the insecurities of those able to afford supplements and excluding those who cannot.

In the developing world, however, the situation is much simpler: sickness and extremes of poverty have long ensured that there is no choice at all for much of the world's population. Something has gone desperately wrong.

Although the concept of food that could meet all our nutritional requirements, act as a preventive agent against illness and alleviate the world's food shortages may seem like a fantasy, it is not so far from the truth as some people may think. In fact, a food with properties very similar to those out-lined above does exist on the earth today – and has done for more than three billion years. It is the oldest life-form on the planet and pre-dates even mankind by more than two billion years. Stone age man knew about it, and the ancient Egyptians, Aztecs, Mayans, Chinese and Ethiopians ate it to supplement their diets.

Today, it is consumed by primitive African tribes, health-conscious Japanese and fashionable Californians. It is the most highly nutritional food on the planet, with an amino acid, vit-amin and mineral profile closely resembling our own. Moreover, it is cheap and easy to grow. It is blue-green algae.

Blue-green algae is the freshwater relative of sea and ocean plankton, although some blue-green algae can grow in sea water. It lies at the very bottom of the planet's food chain: without it, no life would exist – or would ever have existed – on earth. It is composed of simple, monocellular organisms, the precursors of bacteria, which managed to adapt them-selves to the harsh environment of the Earth when it first came into existence.

Floating in the primordial chemical soup that distilled into the world's oceans, seas, rivers and lakes, blue-green algae – or cyanobacteria – absorbed nitrogen from the atmos-phere and, via photosynthesis, produced life-giving carbo-hydrates, proteins, amino acids, vitamins and enzymes. Blue-green algae also released the first oxygen into the atmos-phere which many millions of years later enabled more devel-oped life forms to evolve on dry land. Today, algae is the staple food of most aquatic creatures, from the largest, the great whale, to microscopic pond life.

Having breathed life into the Earth and laid the founda-tions of the planet's ecosystems, blue-green algae is now forging a second revolution across the world. The Japanese, the most health-conscious nation in the world, have carried out extensive research into the health benefits of blue-green algae, and have pioneered its use as a health food supplement. Today, they consume vast quantities of blue-green algae, and their products – including biscuits, pasta, drinks and spreads as well as capsules, tablets and powder – have been eagerly snapped up by Pacific rim populations, including Californians, Australians and New Zealanders and emerging markets in Europe. The annual global market for blue-green algae supplements is now estimated at $1 billion (£650 million).

Although they appear indistinguishable from any other supplement on the shelves in health-food stores, blue-green algae products are already beginning to revolutionize the way we look at the vitamin industry. Unlike other supplements, blue-green algae contains vast reserves of naturally occurring minerals which the body can assimilate very easily.

It has five times more calcium than milk; fifty times more iron than spinach; three times more protein than meat, fish or poultry; and twice as much beta carotene as carrots. It is also one of the few plant sources of vitamin B12, which is usually found in animal tissues – one teaspoon of blue-green algae contains more than double the amount found in a small serving of liver.

Moreover, blue-green algae has no calories, cholesterol or sodium and even contains natural substances which trick the body into thinking it is not hungry. It is a good food source for dieters, vegetarians, athletes, pregnant and nursing mothers, children, the sick and the elderly. Indeed, it has been shown to be remarkably effective in eliminating the symptoms of pre-menstrual syndrome (PMS) and anaemia and also brings extraordinary regeneration of the hair, skin and nails.

It is also a valuable source of amino acids, chelated minerals, trace elements and enzymes that are lacking from modern Western diets. Although we are told that multivitamin supplements are the answer to our nutritional needs, manufacturers of these products omit to tell us that, in the long run, these synthetic preparations may be damaging to our health.

For, unlike the vitamins and minerals that we extract from foods, which are bound to natural food complexes with proteins, carbohydrates and lipids, most supplements are synthetic combinations of isolated vitamins and minerals with an entirely different structure from those found in foods. Put simply, the body cannot recognize these supplements as food and therefore does not absorb them completely.

Scientists have attempted to overcome this problem by devising megadoses, chemical chelators (mimicking the natural binding agents in food) and time-release agents. However, these new-style vitamins are now thought to do more harm than good, as they can interfere with the body's natural systems and chemical balances.

Blue-green algae has been absent from health-food shops for a decade because in the early 1980s it acquired a false reputation as a miracle food for dieters, which was subsequently discredited. In 1981, the US tabloid, the *National Enquirer*, created huge nationwide demand for spirulina when it published reports that US doctors had discovered a remarkable new slimming pill. Demand soon outstripped supply as obese Americans from all over the country tried to get their hands on a pill that would magic away their excess pounds.

Of course, there was a grain of truth behind the disastrous marketing campaign. Scientists have shown that blue-green algae does indeed contain an amino acid called phenylalanine which can act as an effective appetite suppressant. However, this can only help people lose weight if they also adhere to a

low-fat or low-calorie diet. Blue-green algae can help slimmers curb their appetites and maintain blood sugar at a level
that prevents hunger pangs, but it is certainly no substitute for
willpower.

Unfortunately, as demand grew, suppliers were forced to
add bulking agents to eke out the limited supplies of blue-
green algae and this, together with the misleading promise of
a miracle cure, gave the supplement a bad name which
endured for many years.

Blue-green algae also lost favour when scientists reported
that some strains of cyanobacteria are prone to develop potent
toxins which can be fatal to humans. Although this is generally true for cyanobacteria, it is important to point out that the
scientists omitted to say that these toxins only develop in certain climatic conditions, where there is, for example, excess
heat or stagnant water.

All the blue-green algae products available in the shops in
the UK, US, Europe, Asia and Australasia are constantly
monitored for toxins and, so far, none has ever been found in
either Lake Klamath AFA or spirulina. It is thought that the
pure environment and climate (particularly the cold, harsh
winters) of Lake Klamath are instrumental in protecting the
algae and ensuring that only the hardiest and healthiest strains
survive. The artificial conditions under which spirulina is
grown also mitigate against the danger of toxic outbreaks.

Anyone considering taking blue-green algae should, of
course, only use approved and tested products from health-
food shops. Although it is tempting to think that a handful of
algal weed from clean country rivers would be just as effective, it really would be dangerous to consume anything like
this. The carefully controlled growing environments of harvested blue-green algae ensure that only the highest quality
products reach the market.

Over the last decade, scientists across the world have been examining blue-green algae in their labs, extracting different substances from it which have been shown to be remarkably effective in the treatment of conditions such as cancer and AIDS. Extracts of blue-green algae have also been shown to protect laboratory rats and hamsters against cancer, while researchers in the US have found that its sulfolipids have destroyed the HIV virus in laboratory tests.

Although it would be obviously irresponsible to label blue-green algae as a miracle cure for such conditions, scientific studies have shown that it possesses remarkable health-giving properties. As well as building and maintaining health, it is also superb for reducing cholesterol, boosting the immune system and friendly intestinal bacteria, eliminating toxins and treating malnutrition.

Moreover, it has been shown to improve a whole host of conditions: giving relief from physical and mental stress; balancing hormonal cycles; improving the condition of hair, skin and gums; reducing allergic reactions; curbing food cravings; and balancing weight. It also increases vitality, improves memory and heightens mental clarity.

During the last five years, doctors in the US and Europe have been quietly using blue-green algae to relieve symptoms of cancer and AIDS, attributing its remarkable effect to the antioxidant effects of its beta carotene (which deactivates free radicals that damage cells and can cause cancer) and the fact that it builds healthy intestinal lactobacillus, which is known to protect against infection and stimulate the immune system.

Perhaps the most dramatic example of blue-green algae's efficacy can be seen at Chernobyl, in Belarus, where doctors from the Institute of Radiation Medicine have successfully treated children who suffered radiation sickness as a result of the nuclear reactor disaster in 1985. Five grams of spirulina, a blue-green algae, reduced the levels of radioactivity in their urine by 50 per cent as well as improving their general health by providing important extra nutrients. It was also shown to reduce the toxic side-effects of drugs on the liver and kidneys. Since their initial findings, doctors have regularly treated one hundred children every twenty days with blue-green algae.

NASA scientists are also researching the potential of blue-green algae as a food of the future for use on space pro-grammes and even remote stations on different planets. Early in the next century, NASA plans to put a space station into orbit which will be manned by US, Japanese and European astronauts who will be supported by a regenerative life sup-port system. They are particularly interested in its phenome-nal ability to synthesize high quality food efficiently and produce oxygen in environments dominated by toxic gases such as nitrogen and methane.

In another field, genetic researchers are considering the use of algae in gene transfer. Scientists are currently examin-ing the effects of developing algae that will live in the epider-mis of domestic animals (goats, pigs and cattle) which will eventually enable them to live in dry environments with minimal demands for food and water as they learn to photo-synthesize their food from sunlight and oxygen.

Other researchers believe that algae could also be adapted to live in some humans, using protozoa and bacteria that digest cellulose so that they can live in the human gut and convert the material there into sugars, volatile fatty acids and amino acids that can be absorbed and metabolized by man, thus making many inexpensive vegetarian (grass) food sources available to man for food.

Of course, this is a long way off in the future. At present, blue-green algae offers a real solution to our health needs – both for the over-fed nations of the West and the under-fed nations of the developing world. Good health can become our birthright once again if we revert to eating more natural foods and supplementing our diets with superfoods such as blue-green algae. Our future is in our own hands, as this book will explain.

Chapter 1

THE STATE WE'RE IN: THE TWENTIETH-CENTURY HEALTH CRISIS

How blue-green algae can restore world health

If we eat wrongly, no doctor can cure us;
if we eat rightly, no doctor is needed.
Dr Victor G. Rocine, 1930

Food has always been our best medicine. Everything we need to stay healthy can be found in nature's abundant storehouse, including medicines that can heal us should we fall sick. Today, at the end of the twentieth century, those of us who are privileged enough to live in the Western world enjoy higher standards of hygiene than ever before and have unparalleled choice and access to food and excellent health care. Yet, surprisingly, we are among the worst-nourished nations in the world.

The shocking fact is that, even though we do not suffer the famines or food shortages of the undeveloped world, many of us are no better nourished than the severely malnourished peoples of the undeveloped world. As we have become more affluent, we have acquired poor eating habits: we regularly miss meals or eat too fast, which can put a great strain on our gastro-intestinal tract; we eat diets rich in refined sugar, cholesterol and salt (which appeal to our tastebuds) and low in fibre, which puts a strain on the eliminative processes as these types of food remain in the colon for a long time, increasing the risk of a build-up of toxins.

The biggest killers of the Western world – heart disease, digestive disorders, cancer, and other degenerative diseases – are virtually unheard of in rural communities in Africa and India, where the inhabitants subsist on simple diets of vegetables and wholegrains. Scientists have shown that when primitive peoples, such as Eskimos, North American Indians and Aborigines, who had never experienced digestive problems, constipation, tooth decay or even painful childbirth in their own cultures, were fed Western diets, they quickly succumbed to all the problems we experience. We know therefore that diet is largely to blame for heart disease, obesity, tooth decay and some types of cancer.

Western medicine conspires with this great marketing plan. We eat nutrient-starved foods, take vitamin and mineral supplements our bodies cannot fully utilize and, not surprisingly, fall prey to a wide range of illnesses. Instead of teaching us how to get back to basics and really look after ourselves, doctors treat diseases caused by unnatural foods as if they were an inevitable part of life. Millions of pounds are spent each year on drugs to control obesity, heart disease, digestive disorders and cancer. If we stood back for a moment and observed the reasons why chronic illness develops, we could avoid much of this misery.

Diet affects not only our physical, but our mental health. Studies in the US have found evidence that the growth of the fast-food industry correlates with the growth of antisocial behaviour, violence and even murder in the country. According to one study, scientists discovered that when white sugar, fast food and low-nutrient foods were removed from the diets of teenage offenders guilty of violent crime and burglary, and replaced with high quality fruit, vegetables and cereals, there was a 48 per cent decrease in their antisocial behaviour. We now know that junk foods – high fat and high sugar foods, which are low in live enzymes, vitamins and minerals – can cause chronic vitamin deficiencies that interfere with the proper functioning of the brain and upset the nervous system.

The problems with our food

Fifty years ago, most people knew what constituted a good diet and gave it little thought. Today, with the rise of packaged convenience foods, junk food and ready-made meals, whole generations have grown up without understanding even basic nutrition or simple cooking skills. Even though we live much longer and we have a wider range of foods to choose from, a growing number of people are not confident about what they eat and drink.

The reasons for this are many and varied. One is the fact that in the last fifty years our food has become less nutritious, so we have to eat proportionately more to derive an adequate level of vitamins and minerals. As well as this, it has become the norm to eat high fat 'junk' foods, which are packed with empty calories rather than nutrients.

There has also been a revolution in the production and distribution of food. In the last fifty years, food has become a highly profitable industry, controlled as much by scientists and entrepreneurs as farmers. The evidence for this is everywhere to be seen. No longer do we have to wait for the steady march of the seasons to enjoy our favourite foods: in the depths of winter we can enjoy farmed salmon with French beans flown in from Kenya, followed by strawberries from Israel. In summer, we can have winter root vegetables, dates and tangerines.

Not only do we have access to an unparalleled choice in food, but the prices of certain foods that were once considered luxuries – chicken, beef and fish – have also fallen considerably. We do not have to supplement our diets with fruits and vegetables because high-protein foods have become so cheap. This all seems like good news for the shopper, but it actually belies some worrying trends.

The British public is, perhaps, more aware than most people of the dangers lurking in our food. In recent years, we have been exposed to a whole plague of food scares which have made us much more careful about what we eat. The most dramatic of these was the admission in spring 1996 that bovine spongiform encephalopathy (BSE) had been detected in the British dairy herd. The epidemic actually began in 1986, when the Government deregulated the food industry, allowing feed manufacturers more flexibility in developing products for cattle.

Unfortunately, they decided to add cheap offal from sheep to make up the protein content of the feed; by law, they were not obliged to disclose this fact to farmers. Thus, vegetarian animals were fed animal protein, causing a terrible breakdown in the natural order. The feed manufacturers did not eliminate scrapie, a disease similar to BSE, which sheep have carried for centuries in Britain.

Although much of the research has come to light only this year, it appears that, for more than a decade, the public has been at risk from BSE-infected meat used in products such as sausages, pies and pasties. (BSE usually occurs in cows aged three to five, whose meat is used in these products, whereas steak and quality cuts come from two-year-old bullocks.) Scientists have now linked BSE to Creutzfeld-Jakob

Disease (CJD), which affects the brain and central nervous system. There is currently no cure for BSE.

There have been similar scares involving the egg and poultry industry: in the late 1980s, an unusual number of people developed food poisoning from salmonella found in eggs and poultry. When pregnant women suffered miscarriages and young children and old people died as a result of the salmonella outbreak, the Government ordered the destruction of millions of eggs to prevent more tragedies. Again, the public suspected that bad farming practices, such as over-working battery hens, was a contributory factor to the disaster and many people turned to organically farmed or free-range eggs.

Although these scares have done much to raise people's awareness of what we are putting in our mouths, there are more widespread and insidious problems which the general public is not made aware of, for obvious reasons. Chief among these is the startling **lack of nutrients** in our fresh fruit and vegetables. Scientists estimate that in order to get the equivalent iron content from a single bowl of spinach harvested in 1948, we would need to eat seventy-five similar bowls today. They have even discovered in tests that some oranges contain no vitamin C whatsoever.

There is a simple reason for this decline in nutrients – our soil does not contain enough nutrients itself to pass any on to the food that grows in it. Over-cultivation and mass farming methods have left it exhausted. Of course, this did not happen overnight. The decline began fifty years ago, after the end of the Second World War, when farmers were encouraged to use **chemical fertilizers**, made of phosphorus, potassium and nitrate, rather than natural fertilizers such as manure, to maximize their crop yields. In fact, the farmers themselves had been duped as the Government had dumped all their stocks of nitrates, which had been produced for bombs during the war, on to them, without warning them of the long-term effects the chemicals would have on the soil.

In the short term, crops did double and food was plentiful, but the harsh chemicals killed off naturally occurring micro-organisms in the soil which change minerals into organic form so our bodies can absorb them. Since then, farmers have continued to be more interested in quantity – representing profit – than quality. They replace only the bare minimum of nutrients in the soil and prefer to grow hybrid strains, which look good and are easy to harvest and store. On top of this, produce is often harvested long before it is ripe and is packed in cold storage and shipped across the world in order to meet year-round demands.

The result is that, even if we eat the recommended five daily portions of fruit and vegetables, we will not get enough vitamins and minerals to keep us healthy. The only way to ensure that we are getting enough vitamins is to buy organic produce, which, unfortunately, is still prohibitively expensive for most people.

The long-term effect of these practices is that nitrate has now become established in the food chain, especially in vegetables. Although nitrate is not itself toxic, it can produce nitrate, which is found in bacon and ham (where it is used as a preservative), beer and drinking water, and has been linked to 'blue baby syndrome' in infants fed on milk containing high levels of nitrites. Nitrites can also form compounds in the body called nitrosamines and nitrosamides which are powerful carcinogens.

Many scientists and doctors believe that the dearth of vitamins and minerals in our food is an important factor in the growing incidence this century of degenerative diseases, such as cancer. One example of the potentially damaging effect of mineral and vitamin deficiencies that can be traced back to chemical fertilizers is in the depletion of magnesium levels in soil. Magnesium suffers most from the widespread use of chemical fertilizers, with the result that it is now woefully lacking in our soil and in our diet. This has been linked to the growing incidence of cancer and leukaemia in children and adults in the UK. Other deficiencies are linked to the upsurge, particularly among children, of allergies such as asthma, and degenerative diseases such as ME, MS and lupus.

Around 100,000 per cent more chemicals are used on farmland and crops today than in 1945. Scientists estimate that the average person who shops in a regular supermarket and eats fruits and vegetables at each meal will ingest approximately one gallon of **pesticides** each year, even if we wash our produce. Our bodies have no chance to eliminate these poisons, many of which are complex chemicals, which we have simply not evolved to process. Not knowing what to do with them, these toxins are stored in our body tissues and, more damagingly, our vital organs.

In the mid-1960s, the Government introduced laws to restrict the use of some pesticides, including organochlorine compounds such as DDT and DDE. We now know that several pesticides and herbicides can cause cancer and birth defects. Last year, a US court awarded substantial damages to a couple whose child had been born anophthalmic – without eyes – because his mother had been exposed to high levels of the fungicide benlate in the early stages of her pregnancy. Nine Scottish families whose children were born with the same condition, anophthalmia, are now suing Dupont, which manufactures benlate.

Another dangerous chemical is the pesticide daminazide – or alar – which is sprayed on apple trees to make the fruit develop a red colour and fertilize the trees, and which cannot be washed off the fruit. Although it is not widely used in Britain, in the US, alar has been found in apple juice in significant amounts and scientists believed that it could be a factor in the development of cancer.

Not only is the food we eat laden with pesticides and chemicals, we also have to think about the other two fundamental elements of life: the **air** we breathe and the **water** we drink. A hundred years ago, this would have been unthinkable, at least in the countryside, outside the main industrial regions. Now, as we approach the end of the twentieth century, we are subjected to a potent cocktail of poisons in the air, including pesticides from crops, heavy metals from industrial pollution, petroleum and car fumes, which leech precious oxygen from the atmosphere.

It is calculated that Londoners alone breathe in as much as a litre of gaseous heavy metals each year: every litre of London air contains a millionth part heavy metal and, on average, we breathe a million litres each year.

Heavy metals such as mercury and cadmium are released into the atmosphere by industrial plants. Mercury salts, for instance, can be converted by bacteria into toxic organic forms such as methyl mercury which can be absorbed into the food chain. Fish, in particular, can accumulate mercury and cause illness, brain damage and even death when eaten. Cadmium has also been discovered in plants, soil and crops adjacent to smelting works and is common in shellfish, such as crab. This heavy metal can cause kidney damage and high blood pressure.

Although tap water is theoretically safe to drink in Britain, its quality varies from region to region, with some areas having higher levels of fluoride or nitrates. Although disasters involving drinking water are rare – the exception being the Camelford tragedy in Cornwall, when water was poisoned with mercury, resulting in a high incidence of cancer in the local population years later – pollutants do find their way into water. Chemical fertilizers, pesticides, herbicides, industrial chemicals, acid rain and chemically produced oestrogen appear to be finding their way into our water at alarming speed. For this reason, many people prefer to filter water through charcoal or drink bottled mineral water than rely on tap water.

Nutritionists advise us to eat as few refined or processed foods as possible, as many of these contain **additives** – chemicals that have been added either to preserve or sterilize them during the processing. The use of additives is strictly controlled by law. Some additives, such as tartrazine E102 and benzoic acid (E210) can cause allergic reactions in susceptible people and should be avoided.

Sulphur dioxide, which is present as a **preservative** in wine, can trigger asthma attacks. Similarly, antioxidants, such as ascorbic acid, are added to fruit juices to stop them going brown and butylated hydroxytoluene (BHT) and butylated hydroxyanisole (BHA) are added to vegetable oils to stop them going rancid. Some studies have shown that rats fed high quantities of both BHA and BHT are more likely to develop cancer.

Freezing food can also destroy nutrients; vegetables are routinely blanched before freezing, which means that they can lose as much as 25 per cent of their mineral content in the process. Meat and fish are similarly affected: meat loses much of its iron content when it is thawed and fish loses much of its iodine.

Flour-refining has been shown to remove as much as 75 per cent of the natural minerals in the grain as well as much of the vitamin content: the refining process produces bread which will stay fresher longer, but which retains hardly any of the natural goodness of the original grain.

Sugar is present in many foods as a preservative and flavour-enhancer, but it provides what nutritionists term 'empty calories'. The famous naturopath, Dr Paavo Airola, estimated that each person in the West consumes around 125 pounds of sugar every year. Many scientists now believe that sugar – sometimes dubbed the 'white poison' – is so bad for our bodies that, were it man-made, it would be banned as a poison. One of the cumulative effects of excess refined sugar consumption is hypoglycaemia (low blood sugar) which affects as much as 70 per cent of the population.

Artificial sweeteners, such as aspartame, sorbitol and manitol, are best avoided along with sugar as they have been known to cause allergic reactions in some people, including headaches, blurred vision and hyperactivity, although these effects are anecdotal and have not been substantiated in scientific studies.

The environment

The destruction of rainforests and the growing hole in the ozone layer expose us to harmful ultraviolet rays, which some scientists have linked to cancer. **Acid rain** – caused by pollution – destroys naturally occurring minerals in our soil, such as selenium. Worse, environmental disasters, such as the explosion of the nuclear reactor at Chernobyl, Belarus, in 1986 shows how far **radiation contamination** can spread through the atmosphere. More than a decade after the accident, sheep in the Lakeland district of Cumbria still cannot be sold for meat, as the land they graze on is still contaminated by nuclear fallout. In parts of Europe, levels of caesium radionuclides 134 and 137, which can accumulate in the food chain, became so high that produce was banned.

Fish have also become contaminated in seas off parts of Britain, following the dumping of nuclear waste into the sea by nuclear power stations. Although scientists at one stage believed that the waste would be diluted by sea water, it in fact became concentrated in certain areas, which led to the contamination of fish. In 1986, fish caught off the Cumbrian coast near the Sellafield nuclear plant were found to be 200 times more radioactive than those in non-contaminated areas.

Our bodies are exposed to radiation every day. Nuclear plants often have leakages which, although they are nowhere near as big in scale as the Chernobyl disaster, nevertheless can have a damaging cumulative effect through low-level radiation. Radon gas, the radioactive by-product of naturally occurring uranium decay, has also been detected in the atmosphere emanating from gypsum, bricks, concrete or phosphates which contain uranium.

In hospitals, medical equipment, such as X-ray, CAT or mammography scanners, use radiation, while military weapon sites often contain nuclear weapons whose radioactive elements can seep into the atmosphere.

However, probably the most insidious form of radiation sickness can come from smoking cigarettes. Scientists have discovered that cigarette smoke contains the radioactive elements radium-226 and potassium-40 which, when inhaled, expose the smoker to radiation that is hundreds of times greater than any naturally occurring radiation.

The result of being exposed to radioactive particles – whether through smoke, in airborne particles, through nuclear disasters or through food grown in radioactive soil – is the production of free radicals in the body, which disrupt the functions and structures of tissues. Free radicals (which can also occur in the body when it is exposed to pollution, some medical drugs and UV light) destroy lipids, enzymes and proteins and can cause cells to die by disrupting DNA/RNA structure and cell metabolism. In short, they disrupt and deplete the immune system, damaging cells and blood vessels, which can lead to degenerative diseases, such as cancer.

Although nutrition is still a developing science, most experts agree that the level of toxins, chemicals and contaminants in food is greater the higher you eat on the food chain. In simple terms, if you eat fish, you will be exposed to more toxins than if you eat pulses or grains because you will also ingest all the toxins that have accumulated in the bodies of the small fry your fish has eaten, and all the shrimps that the small fry have eaten. Similarly, the meat of sheep or cows that have grazed on land treated with chemicals will have absorbed those chemicals, as well as heavy metals and toxins in air and water, and these will be passed on to the meat-eater. Blue-green algae, however, sits at the very bottom of the food chain.

Stress – the silent destroyer

As well as chemical fertilizers in our soil, pesticides on our crops, additives in our foods, heavy metals in the environment and the dangers of radiation and UVA rays, we also compound the organic problems in our bodies with our frantic lifestyles.

In the 1990s, many women work, leaving them with little time to prepare elaborate meals at home. Supermarkets have recognized this fact of life and have introduced ranges of ready-meals that will appeal to working mothers and single people who do not have the time to cook. Although many of these meals are a marvel of convenience – often delicious as well as easy to prepare – they are often over-processed and not balanced enough in their vitamin, mineral, fat and protein content. They also contain preservatives, colourants and additives, the dangers from which have been outlined above.

Yet scientists say that our busy lifestyles and the growth in environmental pollutants have significantly increased our dietary requirements for certain essential nutrients. So, with the lack of nutrients in modern foods and our reliance on refined foods, we are doubly exposed to the dangers of degenerative disease which can occur when the body is seriously depleted of proper nutrients.

Emotional stress, frustration, high noise levels, anxiety, lack of exercise and oxygen can also cause great stress in the body. Many busy people working in air-conditioned offices are starved of oxygen, which is needed to eliminate toxins from the body. Without oxygen, these toxins can accumulate and lead to degenerative diseases. Emotional stress produces excessive adrenalin which requires oxygen for its metabolism, while physical trauma can reduce circulation and hence oxygen to the cells. When bacterial infections and viruses attack our bodies, immune cells need up to 50 per cent of the body's oxygen to fight the infections satisfactorily.

In summary, stress affects every cell and tissue of the body and, if it becomes chronic, it can impair the effectiveness of the immune system, leaving us exposed to serious illness and affecting the digestive system and hindering the absorption, metabolism and elimination of food.

The vitamin myth

Modern science has, of course, found the ultimate scientific solution for the problems fifty years of chemical tampering have caused in our food. With a brainwave as breathtakingly illogical as their idea to give cattle artificial hormones when they discovered that traces of chemical fertilizers in grass they ate made them sterile, scientists developed artificial vitamins and minerals in laboratories and sold them to us as supplements. These we now take by the ton to compensate for our poor diets.

The question, of course, is why the scientists did not tackle the root of the problem – the dearth of nutrients in our soil. Probably because they realized that such depletion could not be fixed overnight, whereas they could quickly develop and sell vitamin and mineral supplements to a large group of affluent people who were concerned about their health. They spotted a potentially lucrative market and soon, a worldwide industry, worth billions of pounds, was born.

Today, it is as natural for many people to take a handful of vitamin pills as it is to eat a meal. Most health-food stores and pharmacies stock a bewildering range of supplements, some of which can cost tens of pounds. The marketing machine has worked so well that we now have to choose between different tiers of supplements – multi-doses, mega-doses, chelated vitamins and so on. What they do not emphasize, however, is that very few of these supplements bear any resemblance to natural foods. With the exception of fish oils, evening primrose oil, royal jelly, ginseng and some of the newer health 'foods', supplements such as vitamin A, vitamin B12, selenium, zinc, magnesium or potassium, are synthetic.

These supplements do not come from nature, but have been concocted by scientists in laboratories, who either synthesize or isolate them from their natural source using chemical means. The resulting vitamins and minerals are then either pressed into tablets, made into capsules or suspended in a solution. Because they are not in their natural state, the body can only use a proportion of the vitamins and minerals they contain, even though they are formulated to claim 100 per cent of the recommended daily allowance.

In whole, or natural foods, vitamins and minerals are bound to natural food complexes with proteins, carbohydrates and lipids. Held in such a structure, the body can recognize them as food and assimilate them easily. In fact, the body is designed to break down foods and use them according to their complex structure – for instance, certain minerals help the body absorb iron, which is difficult to assimilate when it is isolated in a tablet. No scientist could ever attempt to emulate the complex array of vitamins and minerals in foods, but it is precisely this array which works so well for us.

Scientists attempted to overcome the problem of absorption by developing mega'doses, assuming that more (and more expensive) always means better. However, this approach appears to be flawed because scientists now recognize that the intestines regulate and limit the uptake of vitamins, meaning that any excess will automatically be eliminated rather than stored in the body. Worse, it now appears that if the body begins to rely on mega-dose formulas of supplements, it can become lazy and forget how to extract nutrients efficiently from foods, thereby blocking the body's natural wisdom.

Even cleverer researchers developed chemical chelators, which bind vitamins, transporters and time-release mechanisms, to prevent elimination. Yet the chemicals they used to develop these mechanisms left residues which affected some people adversely. Then, they went one step further, by combining extracted vitamins and minerals with real foods, such as yeast, and proclaiming these were the new generation supplements.

It does not take a genius to recognise this as madness. Yet

so many people have been fooled by the claims of vitamin and mineral supplements. Their great myth and power was that they appeared to hold perfect health in a bottle and, no matter how unbalanced our diet or lifestyle, they could save us. Unfortunately, they may be doing us harm as well as burning a great hole in our pockets.

What we can do about it

Sometimes it is hard to keep abreast of the conflicting advice we are given about nutrition. Nutrition is still a developing science and the tremendous diversity of opinions among nutritionists suggests that we have not yet developed a full understanding of even the basics of nutrition.

Barely a week goes by, it seems, without doctors or scientists completely changing their minds about what is good or bad for us. Once, bread, potatoes, pasta, chocolate and butter were the foods we had to avoid; now we are told that chocolate is good for the brain, red wine is good for the heart and most of our calorie intake should come from bread, pasta and potatoes.

The vast majority of people are, not unnaturally, confused. Some try so hard to eat foods that are perceived as 'healthy' that they miss out on other, equally important foods which may be out of fashion, while others simply give up and eat exactly what they want without even paying lip-service to basic nutritional guidelines. Some people are so confused that they experience panic attacks at the mere mention of food or when it is time to prepare a meal.

It is time to inject a measure of simplicity in our attitudes to food. We must realize that, whatever scientists, nutritionists or doctors say, our bodies have been programmed for thousands of years to deal with natural, whole foods. Every time a chemical is added or a nutrient subtracted from the natural balance, our bodies will suffer. When additives, preservatives, dyes, irradiation and microwaves are added to the equation, the problems are magnified.

Scientists can develop processed foods, genetically engineered and enhanced foods and even totally synthetic chemical 'foods', but it will take thousands more years of evolution for our bodies to cope with such technological advances. In the mean time, our bodies will simply store chemicals they do not recognize or know how to process in tissues and vital organs, causing long-term health problems.

It may seem old-fashioned and retrograde to reject these exciting new advances in food technology, but our health is surely more important than passing fashions. In truth, the marketing machine has worked so well against our instincts that the natural way to eat actually seems outdated and boring. In fact, society is so out of touch with nature that anyone who advocates the most basic, natural foods is dismissed either as a crank or hopelessly idealistic. Nothing could be further from the truth.

To maintain good health, we need to ensure our bodies get fresh air, pure water, a moderate amount of exercise, and certain nutrients. These simple requirements are, as we have discovered, difficult to obtain, but regular visits out of cities to the coast or countryside, drinking mineral or filtered water and, where possible, eating an organic or whole-food diet can achieve most of them. On a very basic level, our bodies are machines that need proteins, minerals, vitamins and energy foods, such as carbohydrates and fibre, to keep them running smoothly.

Proteins, which can be obtained from meat, fish, poultry, eggs and nuts, are made up of amino acids – the building blocks of life. Amino acids comprise 90 per cent of the haemoglobin in our bodies and therefore form the core of the immune system. There are twenty-two amino acids, eight of which are essential for our survival and must be obtained daily from our food as they cannot be stored in the body. Without adequate supplies of amino acids, health cannot be maintained and the body begins to cannibalize tissues in a desperate search for them, causing ageing, memory loss, low mental awareness and depression. Deficiencies have also been linked to more serious medical conditions, including schizophrenia, heart disease, cancer and impotence.

We also need regular quantities of **vitamins** (found in fruits, vegetables and cereals) in our diets for normal growth, vitality and maintenance of health. Vitamins do not provide energy or build the body, as carbohydrates and proteins do, but they are needed for transforming our food into energy. The human body cannot store vitamins for long, so a regular intake is required. Vitamins cannot function without minerals, which are found in traces in many foods. In fact, all nutrients require minerals as the catalyst for activity. A severe deficiency of any one mineral can seriously disrupt the metabolic chain in the body, rendering other nutrients ineffective. This is why it is so important to eat a wide range of foods and a balanced diet.

Finally, **antioxidants**, such as the naturally occurring beta carotene are vital to boost oxygen levels in the body and prevent toxic build-ups. When oxygen levels are low, the body cannot fight infections or deal with toxins and it becomes a breeding ground for degenerative diseases. Studies over the last twenty-five years have shown that people who consume a higher than average amount of beta carotene suffer less cancers of the lung, stomach, colon, bladder, uterus ovaries and skin.

Health is not our birthright; but everyone can maximize their chances of good health by taking responsibility for their diet and lifestyle. This book will outline a new path to health, using unadulterated natural foods, common sense, and a new generation of true 'wholefoods' which can make up for the inadequacies of our depleted storehouse.

Blue–green algae is foremost among these foods, as its nutritional profile is unmatched, weight for weight, by any other food on the planet. It contains around 60 per cent high quality protein and its amino acid profile almost exactly matches the need of the human body in a form that is almost 100 per cent bioassimilable.

Moreover, blue–green algae contains a little of nearly all the vitamins and minerals needed by the body in organic form, including valuable trace minerals which cannot be found in other foods. It also has active enzymes which enable the body to absorb it without drawing on the body's own enzyme reserves. Its high content of beta carotene, chlorophyll and antioxidant pigments boosts the immune system, oxygenates the body and regenerates and purifies the blood.

Of course, blue–green algae will seem like a strange form of nutrition to some people. Its bright blue–green colour and strong smell will not appeal to everyone, but the parlous state of our food should be a warning that it is time for us to rethink our attitudes to food. If we can learn to appreciate simple, wholesome foods like blue–green algae, which are good for us, even if they do not immediately appeal to our sense of taste and smell, then we will have taken the first step back to assuming responsibility for our health.

Like any habit, good ones can also stick and our reward from blue–green algae is more energy, increased emotional stability, vibrant, glowing health and some peace of mind in a mad, mad world.

Chapter 2

BLUE-GREEN ALGAE: OUR ANCESTOR AND FRIEND

The simple organism that revolutionized the planet

Healing is a matter of time, but it is also sometimes a matter of opportunity.

Hippocrates

As we stand on the threshold of a new millennium, it is worth pausing for a moment to consider how far we have evolved and what we have become. As we saw in the preceding chapter, during the last hundred years our food has become less natural, our environment more polluted and our lives more stressful than ever before in our history.

However, lest we we begin to think that the future is all doom and gloom, there is some good news as far as our health is concerned. In the last five years, a new generation of wholefoods has emerged which promises to revolutionize the way we look at nutrition. They represent a backlash against the horde of synthetic vitamins and minerals which dominate the shelves in pharmacies and health-food stores and demand exorbitant prices. The new foods are high-potency foods, which occur naturally and include ginseng, bee pollen, wheat grass, barley essence and royal jelly.

Head and shoulders above these foods – as far as its nutritional profile is concerned – is blue-green algae, the oldest life-form on the planet. This micro algae, which grows in both sea water and fresh water, was the first life-form to colonize the earth 3½ billion years ago and is the precursor of all plants and animals. It has been used down the centuries for both its nutritional and healing properties, but has been all but forgotten in the twentieth century. Now, in the very nick of time, we have woken up to its potential once more.

In this chapter, we shall examine how blue-green algae, a simple organism which has been on Earth since the beginning of time, can save us from our headlong and seemingly inexorable descent into ill health.

Wisdom of blue-green algae

Blue-green algae (or cyanobacteria) has been extraordinarily successful over the last 3½ billion years: it evolved quickly, colonizing the planet and mastering harsh and varied environments; it outwitted competitors, and physical and chemical changes without too much difficulty. In fact, it is true to say that blue-green algae is nothing less than an expert master of survival – it has learnt to produce the right kind of molecules and how to instantly modify or change them, and also how to produce the correct enzymes and vitamins and the proper amino acids in the precise amounts to keep itself healthy.

It has also learnt which pigments to produce and use in various light situations, which would enable it to produce the food it needs, and how to take nitrogen from the air and water and minerals in just the right amount from the water.

Now at last we too have woken up to its potential and the possibilities of survival it can offer us – in terms of improved health and well-being – in the twenty-first century and beyond. Now, more than ever before, we need new, friendly bacteria, such as blue-green algae, to give us protection from environmental toxins, which have only recently been introduced on Earth – man-made electromagnetic radiation, radiation from nuclear plants and toxic chemicals including pesticides, petroleum products and synthetic drugs.

We also need protection from rival, destructive pathenogenic bacteria, which use their incredible survival mechanism to create enzymes that neutralize the drugs we use to kill them. For example, by the late 1950s, because of the over-use of antibiotics in humans and in commercial beef and poultry, certain strains of antibiotic-resistant bacteria began to show up.

These smart, pathenogenic bacteria developed enzymes to digest the drugs, whereas the not-so-smart, weaker bacteria succumbed to the drugs. This resulted in new and deadly drug-resistant bacteria, including certain strains of staphylococcus, syphilis and shigellae. Hospitals in the US and Japan soon reported the same drug-resistant strain, as if these bacteria knew how to develop and share information both simultaneously and globally.

Instead of taking synthetic drugs, which pathogenic bacteria can outwit, it is time for us to play these dangerous bacteria at their own game by eating friendly bacteria such as blue-green algae, which has survival information encoded within its structure and which can fight these deadly new strains of bacteria on our behalf. Blue-green algae has the power not only to nourish us, but to transmit information on healing, survival and environmental protection which it has acquired over countless millennia.

Many nutritionists and some doctors believe that blue-green algae has its own wisdom encoded in its DNA which enables it to act as an intelligent force for healing. It has a glycolipoprotein cell membrane, which can be very easily absorbed by the body – even into the brain – in its natural form. Some nutritionists maintain that this enables blue-green algae's DNA to penetrate our own cellular blueprint, or DNA, read it and direct its healing power to whichever part of the body, mind – or even emotions – that need it. This we shall explore in the following chapters.

What is blue-green algae?

Blue-green algae, also known as cyanobacteria, is a non-flowering aquatic plant related to plankton, seaweed, kelp and ordinary pond slime. Micro-algae grow wherever there is water and sunlight: on land, in soil, on trees, on the surfaces of rocks, in hot springs, in snow and in every river, stream, lake, ocean and sea. They also float in the air and grow in the fur of terrestrial animals and on the skins of sea creatures. Carried in this way by the air, animals, insects or birds, they can travel great distances across the land and sea.

As micro-algae are constantly evolving into new species, they find new and varied habitats all the time. Micro-algae can survive extremes both of cold and heat, living in glaciers and in thermal springs, such as the famous 'Paint Pot' springs in Yellowstone National Park in the US (named after the different colours algae lends to the waters).

According to William Barry, an American expert on algae:

> *They [algae] can double their population every 20 minutes and the results of this can be spectacular, as, for example, when hundreds of square miles of the ocean are turned crim-*

*son by red tide algae or are lit up by miles of bioluminescent
algae, or are made to glow by phosphorescent algae, all in a
matter of hours.*

The Astonishing, Magnificent, Delightful Algae

As Dr Barry indicates, there are many different species of algae
in the world. Some scientists estimate the number of species to
be 50,000. They can range in size from huge ocean kelps,
which can grow as large as sixty metres in length, to micro-
scopically small organisms. Freshwater species are thought to
be much older than seawater algae. They are mostly classified
by colour – the blue-greens, greens, browns, goldens and reds.
The different colours represent the algae's ability to absorb different wavelengths of light, with blue-green algae being able
to absorb the broadest spectrum of light.

Algae perform several very important functions in the
ecosystem. First, they provide food for a vast number of creatures in the world, from tiny insects on land to the great
whale, the largest creature on Earth. Second, they 'fix' the gas
nitrogen from the air or water and act as a natural fertilizer,
enriching soil quality and contributing vital minerals to water.
Third, and most important, they provide 90 per cent of the
oxygen on the planet, with trees and plants contributing the
remaining 10 per cent.

Scientists have described algae as 'the Earth's lungs'
because they estimate that they release 330 billion tonnes of
oxygen into the atmosphere each year. They also protect
against global warming because they absorb dangerous gases,
such as carbon monoxide, which are contributing to the
'greenhouse effect'. Ocean algae are particularly useful in this
respect because these species produce a chemical called
diethyl-sulfonio-propionate which protects them from salt

and which they release into the atmosphere when they die. This release produces another chemical, diethyl sulfide, which scientists believe helps to create clouds, cooling the atmosphere further.

It is not difficult to understand how influential algae are in our ecosystem when you consider that some algal blooms can cover thousands of square miles of the ocean, giving the Earth its distinctive blue-green colour when viewed from outer space.

Earth's first revolutionaries

Blue-green algae holds a special place in our history, as it was the first life-form to colonize the Earth more than 3½ billion years ago. It has survived, virtually unchanged since then, sitting at the very bottom of the evolutionary chain yet, as we have seen, supporting and regulating the Earth's ecosystem.

As far as scientists can tell, the Earth was born around 4½ billion years ago. During its first billion years, after the rocks cooled, heavy rains fell on the Earth creating seas, rivers and vast oceans and dissolving the minerals in the rocks to form soil. The rivers washed minerals and chemicals into the seas and oceans, which were soon brimming with elements such as iron and compounds such as sodium chloride (salt). These substances stole any molecules of oxygen in the atmosphere in order to keep themselves stable, thus preventing life from evolving on Earth.

Countless millennia later, the atmosphere was little more than a primordial soup of minerals, acids, gases and salts which was heated in the warm air and which condensed, eventually, into microbes and bacteria. The Earth was also extremely radioactive.

According to James Lovelock in his book, *The Ages of Gaia*, the Earth was a dead planet whose atmosphere was in an 'abiological steady state'. By this he means that all the chemical components that were needed to create and sustain life were present on the surface of the Earth – amino acids, sugars and nucleosides – but there was one vital element missing: oxygen.

By a quirk of fate or chemistry, blue-green algae suddenly appeared. We know it consisted of simple, one-celled (monocellular) organisms which floated on the surface of bodies of water. Indeed, sedimentary rocks in the Transvaal and in Australia, formed 3½ billion years ago, show fossils of these organisms, which are remarkably similar to blue-green algae we can see in lakes and rivers today.

Cyanobacteria evolved during the Archaean Age of the Earth's history. These hardy cells adapted to the extremes of heat and radioactivity in the Earth's harsh atmosphere and set in motion the entire evolutionary process which has continued until today and which we ourselves are part of. At first, cyanobacteria fed on the abundant chemicals in the water. Later, when some of these chemicals became scarce, they took a remarkable evolutionary leap and learned how to tap the one inexhaustible supply of energy on Earth: sunlight.

This was a remarkable feat in itself, but far more significant was one of the by-products of this action: oxygen. As blue-green algae used solar energy to make organic compounds, they drew on carbon dioxide and broke it down, to release oxygen back into the atmosphere. This was the single most important event in the history of the Earth, for, without oxygen, the planet could never have sustained any evolved form of life.

From that point onwards, life was no longer at the mercy

of the environment. Rather, the potential was there for life to control the atmosphere. For a billion years, blue-green algae dominated the Earth, absorbing poisonous gases and using light, warmth and water to create proteins, carbohydrates, vitamins, minerals and enzymes from which primitive life-forms began to assemble themselves. Over the next three billion years, it released enough oxygen into the atmosphere to create an 'oxic' ecosystem – one that could support more sophisticated forms of life.

According to James Lovelock (Ibid.):

> *I suspect that the origin of Gaia [the Earth as a self-regulating organism] was separate from the origin of life. Gaia did not awaken until bacteria had already colonised most of the planet. Once awake, planetary life would assiduously and incessantly resist changes that might be adverse, and act so as to keep the planet fit for life.*

The creation of food from sunlight is called photosynthesis and cyanobacteria were the first life-forms to develop this remarkable facility. Today, plants still depend on this skill, which they inherited billions of years ago from blue-green algae. In fact, cyanobacteria are so ancient that they straddle the evolutionary fork between bacteria, plants and animals. Being the ancient ancestors of all three kingdoms, blue-green algae shares many characteristics of the three life-forms.

Like bacteria, blue-green algae has remarkable adaptability and can exchange genetic information between cells. Like plants, it uses photosynthesis to produce food and chlorophyll; and, like animals, it has a digestible cell wall that our bodies can assimilate as food.

Cyanobacteria singlehandedly ushered in the next era in the Earth's history, the Proterozoic era, which occurred around 2½ billion years ago. This was the era when oxygen became the predominant gas in the atmosphere and a new form of life – the eukaryotes, from which we are descended – emerged. Eukaryotes were multi-cellular organisms, large groups of cells from which both plants and animals evolved. These cells began life as groups of bacteria, like cyanobacteria, which once moved freely but at some stage became enclosed in a membrane of one of them.

Blue-green algae continued to flourish on land and in water after the eukaryotes appeared, acting as food and still regulating the atmosphere. Then, around 600 million years ago, a bigger organism emerged, which grew into many and varied life-forms. Soon, plants emerged, which could stand erect and draw water and minerals from long roots in the soil and creatures which could travel on land, through the air and in water. This period is called the Phanerozoic and continues today.

Food of the gods

Scientists and nutritionists are using numerous sophisticated techniques to prove the medical and nutritional benefits of blue-green algae. We know that certain extracts are particularly effective in relieving some of the conditions associated with chronic fatigue syndrome, AIDS and cancer. We also know that it can gently and effectively reverse chronic cases of malnutrition and can raise general levels of health in people who are run-down or stressed.

Like many natural foods, however, which we are just beginning to rediscover now that science has finally given them an official sanction, blue-green algae has been enjoyed by ancient civilizations for hundreds of thousands of years. They recognized its extraordinary value for millennia, even if they did not have the benefit of science to prove why it was good for them. With simple wisdom and intuition, they incorporated it into their diets and enjoyed its benefits for generations.

Blue-green algae was known to prehistoric cave dwellers and was a very important source of nutrition. The ancient Egyptians are also known to have consumed algae and Oriental herbalists used it for thousands of years to treat vitamin deficiencies and digestive disorders. It continues to be used widely in the Far East – 300,000 tonnes are consumed in Japan alone each year – and it is only in the last fifty years that it has fallen out of favour in the West. In Europe, the Celts and Vikings, amongst others, consumed algae for hundreds of years.

There are many historical references to the use of algae as a foodstuff in literature. Most important is perhaps the Old Testament book of Exodus, where the starving **Israelites** found a flake-like foodstuff lying on the rocks in the early morning. Believing this was a sign from God, they gave thanks for this 'manna from heaven', which saved them from certain death in the desert. The Israelites described the food as 'tasting like wafers made from honey'.

Scientists now think that the manna they referred to is a form of dried blue-green algae which can survive and lie dormant in the sun-baked deserts of the Middle East. Certain species of algae can survive in the desert even when their pond habitats evaporate and can dry on to rocks. When the algae reaches such a high temperature, the protein is turned into polysaccharide sugars which give it a white, frosted colour and an intensely sweet flavour.

We know from contemporary accounts that blue-green algae, which grew wild in the salt lakes of central Mexico, was highly prized by the **Aztecs**. In fact, archaeologists and anthropologists now acknowledge that the algae was the key to the Aztecs' remarkable civilization. The Aztecs were fierce warriors who conquered much of the Yucatan peninsula, building vast temples and palaces and nurturing a sophisticated culture of art, philosophy and mathematics. They were also skilled craftsmen and artists, weaving magnificent cloths and making highly intricate jewellery and carvings.

Yet archaeologists have long wondered how such a thriving civilization could exist on the meagre food the region supplied, as there was no evidence of the Aztecs keeping domestic animals for food. Cattle, sheep and horses were introduced by the Spanish conquistadores in 1519. Some anthropologists have speculated that since human sacrifice and ritual cannibalism were part of the Aztec culture, human flesh was their main source of protein. Yet we now know that human flesh has very few nutrients, particularly B vitamins, and is notoriously lacking in protein.

It was the Spanish chronicler, Bernal Diaz del Castillo, who travelled with the Spanish commander, Hernán Cortés, to Mexico, who unconsciously held the key to the Aztecs' secret strength. In his dispatches back to the King of Spain, he described the crowded markets in Mexico city, which sold everything from ceramic earthenware, to food, jewellery and animals. One commodity caught his eye because it seemed to be attracting so much attention among the locals. It was called 'tecuitlatl', which means stone excrement in the Aztec language, and consisted of small flat green cakes, which the Spanish described equally unpoetically as 'green mud'. The conquistadores never acquired a taste for tecuitlatl, but for the Aztecs, it was the most important food in their diet.

Contemporary accounts report that the Aztec king, Montezuma, loved to eat fish, but the closest sea to Mexico City was the Gulf of Mexico, around 180 miles away. His court instructed marathon runners to run in relays to the coast to bring fresh fish to Montezuma. The athletes were specially trained and could each run up to a hundred miles a day. For this, they needed a good source of protein – spirulina. Each runner carried small bags of spirulina on their marathons, which they occasionally took to sustain them.

The Aztecs harvested blue-green algae from Lake Texcoco in the Teotihuacan Valley, where Mexico City stands today. They collected it in fine mesh nets and piled it into their canoes. On shore, they patted it into flat cakes and let it dry in the sun. Locals would then buy the cakes and bake it into bread, mix it with grain dishes and add it to sauces.

The Spanish did not appreciate the importance of blue-green algae in the Aztecs' diet, nor did they appreciate the sophisticated technology of the floating gardens – chinampas – on their lakes, where they cultivated vegetables on algal mats. Not realizing that algae could produce more protein than the land could ever yield, they set about draining the great lakes to provide fertile land for their cattle, sheep and crops. Algae is mentioned by Spanish chroniclers until the end of the sixteenth century, but then all references die out. Once the lakes were drained, blue-green algae was not harvested for more than 400 years in Mexico.

Today, where parts of the original lakes remain, there are still traces of blue-green algae. Although most of Lake Texcoco is gone, algae, particularly spirulina, is still farmed in Mexico. This came about by accident, when a company, Sosa Texcoco, set up a plant to extract sodium carbonate from the lake and discovered that blue-green algae was clogging up the machinery. The distillation plants had, in fact, provided the ideal growing conditions for spirulina and the company quickly noted the market potential of spirulina and set up farms to cultivate the food. Today, the company harvests between one and two tonnes of spirulina, most of which is exported to Japan, the world's largest market for blue-green algae.

It is possible that the other great Meso-American civilization – the **Mayans** – also relied on blue-green algae as a source of nutrition. The Mayans, whose population reached more than two million at the height of its civilization between 300 and 900 AD, lived a rather precarious existence in the jungles of the Yucatan Peninsula. The environment was not suited to intensive farming, so the Mayans developed a system of shifting agriculture, whereby they would clear a patch of land in the jungle and farm it for a couple of years before moving on to a new location.

There is evidence that the Mayans cultivated blue-green algae in a network of waterways linking the jungle clearings to provide food for their people and animals. Mexican archaeologists have discovered artificial ponds for growing the algae linked by waterways, which they believe were for cultivating algae rather than for irrigation purposes, as the annual rainfall in the jungle was high enough to sustain crops.

Closer to home, in **Europe**, algae has been used for centuries both as a food source for humans and animals and as a fertilizer. The most popular form of algae in Europe has been kelp, a word which originally referred to the burned ash of brown algae, and which has been used for centuries as a source of salt, iodine and soda. Kelp also contains potash and, when properly processed, will yield tar, ammonia and charcoal, all of which proved vital for household use.

Along the Pacific coast of North America and Canada, other local algae were harvested and used: similarly, China,

South America and the Philippines have all recognized the importance of algae. One of the most original uses for blue-green algae was discovered by accident by a tenth-century monk, Khong Minh Khong, in **Vietnam**. He discovered that rice was much more productive when a water fern, azolla, was planted in the paddy along with the rice plant. Soon, the paddies yielded four times as much rice as before, and the villagers praised him for ensuring that they never again went without food. After the monk's death, they build shrines and temples to him in recognition of his gift to them.

The Vietnamese used this secret for hundreds of years to increase their rice yields. No one knew why azolla was so beneficial to the rice, but they continued to use it, saving many hundreds of thousands of people from starvation. It was only during this century that scientists discovered that azolla was so effective because blue-green algae lived on the fern and fixed nitrogen to it, thereby acting as a powerful natural fertilizer.

Today, in the twentieth century, blue-green algae still has an important place in the diets of both primitive and highly advanced peoples. Although its use has declined spectacularly in the West, particularly in Europe and North America, it is still highly prized in Africa and the Far East.

Spirulina, a species of blue-green algae, has been eaten for centuries by the **Kanembu** people who live along the shores of Lake Chad in central Africa. In 1940, a French phycologist (algae expert) called Dangeard, who travelled to Lake Chad, discovered that blue-green algae was the staple food in Chad. He also discovered that blue-green algae was present in other lakes in Africa, particularly in Lake Nakuru in Kenya's Rift Valley, where thousands of flamingoes subsisted on the algae.

Another researcher, Jean Leonard, a Belgian botanist, also noticed the Kanembus' preoccupation with algae. Like Diaz in Mexico, Leonard noticed that locals at native markets in Ndjamena were eager to buy small green cakes of algae, called Dihé. Leonard traced Dihé's route back to Lake Chad, where he watched the Kanembu women wade into the water, trailing finely woven baskets behind them. They skimmed the surface of the lake to collect the algae, which had been blown by desert winds to the shore and formed into thick mats. Next, they transferred the green sludge into clay pots and took it back to land, where they drained it through cloth to remove excess water and spread it out to dry on the sand. When dry like a biscuit, the women could cut it into small cakes and transport it to market.

The Kanembu people eat Dihé in three-quarters of their meals. They crumble it into tomato and pepper sauces which is then poured over millet, fish or beans. In times of famine, it is a crucial part of the Kanembu diet. Leonard discovered that Kanembu children who were fed the algae showed no signs of the malnutrition that is common among other African tribes. Dihé is also regarded as a powerful talisman by pregnant Kanembu women, who believe that its green'blue colour will protect their unborn children from the eyes of evil spirits and sorcerers.

A world away, in **Japan**, the most health-conscious nation on earth, blue-green algae has long been regarded as the ultimate health food. The Japanese were probably first introduced to the benefits of algae by the Chinese, who have used it for more than 4000 years as a food, a powerful healing agent and a potent aphrodisiac. Today, the Japanese consume more than 300,000 pounds of blue-green algae each year. Japanese scientist Hiroshi Nakamura is one of the world's leading experts on blue-green algae and helped found a micro-algae institute in Tokyo which is dedicated to scientific research on the food.

Although algae was considered as a useful source of food during the war years, when food was rationed, it never took off in Europe. After the war, it fell into oblivion as the agricultural boom of the 1950s and 1960s produced cheap and plentiful food. New farming techniques increased crop yields and before long there was enough high-protein food available without having to resort to foods like algae.

Instead, algae was used in the food and manufacturing industries and as animal feed and fertilizers. Every day, we consume algae in different forms – extracts of algae are used to thicken soups, sauces and cream, and to give peanut butter texture and ice-cream its texture and gloss.

In the textile industry, different algal extracts are used to strengthen fine wools and rayons and to make fine surgical gauze which can be left to dissolve in wounds. Paint and paper also get their gloss and finish from algal products, and it is used to make the coatings of capsules and pills.

Extracts of algae also go into the manufacture of cosmetics such as lipsticks, body oils and soaps, shaving creams and deodorants. They are used in other myriad forms, as gelling agents in confectionery and for dental impressions, pesticide sprays, laxatives, adhesives and in the brewing, canning and tanning industries.

However useful it may be in all these industries, blue-green algae is now being recognized as a source of pure and uncontaminated protein, nutrients and vitamins. As the previous chapter shows, there are very few foods which we can rely on in the modern world to provide us with high levels of nutrients. And, as the world becomes ever more stressful, we need more and more vitamins, minerals and nutrients simply to survive.

Where better to look, then, but at the oldest form of life on Earth? Blue-green algae has been sitting patiently at the bottom of our food chain for millennia, silently supporting our ecosystem and regulating our environment in the face of massive pollution and destruction. It has been waiting for us to wake up to its potential and come to our senses. Whatever scientists might say as they genetically engineer ever more sophisticated strains of foods and breeds of animals, technology cannot compete with nature in its simplicity and perfection.

There is no other food on Earth which is purer or better designed to meet all our nutritional needs. It has more protein, iron and nutrients, gram per gram, than any other food in the world. It sustains life on Earth, from the largest whale to the tiniest insect, and will reproduce itself according to demand. It is cheap, easily cultivated and harvested and provides almost exactly the same amino acid profile as that of our own bodies.

So, on the eve of the new millennium, what do we have to look forward to? The Earth is straining under the demands we are making of it: resources are stretched to the limit as the population continues to grow and the destruction of the rainforests is taking its terrible revenge in wild fluctuations in our climate. Yet, even though it is poised on the brink of catastrophe, somehow the Earth manages to maintain its balance. Much credit for this is due to the constant support of algae, which continue quietly to absorb noxious gases from the atmosphere and release oxygen for us to breathe.

If the human race did push the Earth beyond its limits of endurance, one thing is certain: even if we destroyed ourselves, we could never destroy blue-green algae, which could survive even a nuclear holocaust. Cyanobacteria could survive even the harshest environments – they have done so already, surviving the unimaginably high levels of radiation that existed when the Earth was born. If we destroyed the world, it would be the end of the human race, but blue-green algae would simply adapt to the new environment – and the entire evolutionary cycle would, presumably, recommence.

Blue-green algae has been with us since the dawn of time; without it, we could not have even come into existence and without its continuing help, we would not have enough oxygen to survive for any length of time on Earth. What's more, it has not changed significantly in 3½ billion years. It is so simple in biological terms that it can concentrate completely on manufacturing food. There is no other food on Earth which is so natural; it is our own ancestor and best friend – who, then, would better understand what we need for our survival?

Chapter 3

TWENTY-FIRST-CENTURY NUTRITION: NATURE'S PERFECT SUPERFOOD

Why blue-green algae offers ultimate nutrition

Man alone tries to cook and change his food . . . it is man alone who is subject to the most health trouble . . . The reason is that man does not like to partake of food as God created it.

Sai Baba

There are thousands of species of blue-green algae, but two stand out from the rest because of their spectacularly impressive nutritional profiles. They are *Spirulina platensis* (spirulina), which is cultivated in alkaline lakes throughout the world, including Mexico, New Zealand, Thailand, India, Japan and the US, and *Afanizomenon flos-aquae* (AFA), a wild, freshwater algae which grows predominantly in the northern hemisphere, most notably in the US.

Both share a remarkable nutritional profile, including a high protein content, iron, vitamins, minerals, beta carotene and lipids. Both have, not surprisingly, become popular health supplements – although, technically, each is a complete food rather than a supplement – among health-conscious people around the world.

This chapter will examine in detail the nutritional

content of blue-green algae and look at the way each of its elements – amino acids, proteins, vitamins, minerals and antioxidants – work on the body and how vital they are for the maintenance of good health.

Microalgae have been used as a food source for humans for thousands of years. AFA, chlorella and spirulina are micro-organisms that have drawn attention recently as good sources of high-quality proteins, vitamins, lipids, fine chemicals, glycolipids and sulfolipids. Other genus/species are also being investigated, namely *Porphyridium* and *Dunaliella*.

However, as more and more research is carried out on the two species, a pattern is emerging about the different benefits of each, although they share many of the same characteristics. In simple terms, **spirulina** appears to have a slightly more powerful effect on the body, boosting healing powers and fighting sickness and infection, whereas **AFA** seems to be emerging as a food that will nourish the brain, lifting depression, stimulating motivation and healing the emotions. (This is discussed more fully in Chapter 7.)

Some people tolerate sea water algae better than fresh water algae. Try both separately to see the benefits of each. If you have problems with mental or memory matters, try Klamath Blue Lake first. If you are a smoker and are interested in the antioxidant powers of GLA/beta carotene, try sea spirulina first.

Wild blue-green algae contains a soft cell wall, unlike chlorella and other algae: this feature makes it much easier to digest than cultivated algae – AFA is 95 per cent assimilable, whereas spirulina is 80–90 per cent. Also, wild algae would appear to be better for the mind/emotions, while spirulina is marginally better for nourishing and building the body. Both forms of blue-green algae, however, are among the most powerful healing and cleansing foods in the world.

Today, there are many different kinds of blue-green algae products available in health-food stores and specialist outlets. They range from concentrated liquid algae and freeze-dried or flash-dried powder to capsules, crystals, flakes and tablets to snacks including algae bars, spreads and pasta.

Although these products have long been available in Japan, Mexico and the US, they have only really started to appear in the shops in the UK and continental Europe over the last five years. While blue-green algae is used mainly in specially enriched tonics for women, children and the elderly in the Far East, spirulina is baked into biscuits and crisps in Mexico and Brazil, and New Zealand and Australia market spirulina-based ice-creams and milk shakes. Sweden has spirulina-enriched bread.

In the UK, possibly the most innovative market of all, a whole range of specialist products has been devised using blue-green algae. They include specially formulated drinks for athletes to increase energy and boost performance, and combined supplements to reduce fatigue, PMS and offer antioxidant protection. One British company, AquaSource, markets a particularly effective range of slimming products using AFA which includes a carefully balanced meal-replacement drink in vanilla, banana and strawberry flavours. Many slimmers have used these products successfully to lighten their appetites and lose weight.

How blue-green algae can boost your health

Unlike vitamin and mineral supplements, which attempt to make up for deficiencies in the body, spirulina and AFA offer a perfectly formulated level of nutrition that stimulates the body's systems to work more efficiently, so we tend to absorb more vitamins and minerals from other foods when we eat.

Both spirulina and AFA contain all eight essential and ten non-essential amino acids, which are the building blocks of life. They also have a broad spectrum of vitamins, twenty-seven essential elements or minerals and at least eleven pigments. Blue-green algae is also unusual in the fact that, unlike other algae, it has digestible cell walls, which means that the nutrients are dispersed throughout the organism. In plants, the nutrients are often confined within a membrane, or cell wall, which can be difficult for the body to digest.

Blue-green algae also contains as much as 60 per cent pure protein. Most importantly, its proteins are glycoproteins, as opposed to lipoproteins, which are found in most vegetable matter and beet. In glycoproteins, where the glucose molecule is already attached to the amino acid molecule, the human body's natural process of converting protein into glucose has already begun. As a result, the nutritional contents of algae are highly assimilable and more readily available to the body than most other foods.

Who can benefit from blue-green algae?

People on restricted diets

Anyone who is sick or on a restricted diet, due to diabetes, hypertension, heart disease or allergies, will find that blue-green algae can give a broad range of vitamins and minerals that may otherwise be missing from their diet. Moreover, only small quantities of blue-green algae are needed to provide good nutrition. For anyone taking prescription drugs, algae can act as a powerful detoxifying agent.

Middle age/elderly

A 1988 survey of spirulina customers in Japan were found to be over fifty and 57 per cent of these to be women. Many take it for a particular reason, such as constipation; others because it is a good supplement which can increase energy, vitality and mental alertness.

Children/nursing mothers

Blue-green algae is a useful supplement for children who are fussy eaters and can also have a calming effect on hyperactive children. For pregnant and lactating women, who need extra protein and iron without the extra fat and carbohydrates, it is also a very good supplement. In fact, spirulina is specifically promoted as a vital food for nursing mothers in Vietnam and India.

Vegetarians

Those who avoid meat can derive many important health benefits, but only if they are careful to eat a balanced diet. Meat is, after all, a very easy way of consuming many other major nutrients, including B12 and protein. At least two of the better vegetarian protein sources can be toxic – soya beans and red kidney beans – if they are not prepared properly.

A major concern for anyone on a vegetarian diet is whether or not they are getting enough B12. This is an important consideration for two reasons: meat, dairy products and eggs supply most of the vitamin B12 in the average diet and deficiency can lead to nerve degenerative and death. Fortunately, major studies have found that B12 deficiency is quite rare among vegetarians because our mouths and intestinal bacteria produce this vitamin.

In some individuals, however, the mechanisms of production and absorption are not very efficient. To be on the safe side, all vegetarians should take either B12 supplements or preferably eat algae, which, recent research shows, is by far the richest wholefood source. It is also in a form that the body can easily use.

People who work hard and play hard

Many Japanese businessmen take spirulina with water after a hard night's drinking session. The water is essential for rehydration after alcohol, and blue-green algae supplies protein, vitamins and minerals to rebuild the body's depleted nutrients and help with the morning-after feeling.

Athletes

Athletes need extra nutrition to make up for the energy they expend during vigorous bouts of exercise and training schedules. Blue-green algae is a concentrated source of protein and nutrients that contains very few calories and little fat, meaning that it can be taken to supply energy in the minutes before exercise without impairing performance. (See Chapter 6 for more on athletes.)

Spirulina and AFA

Spirulina

Although spirulina has been cultivated in Mexico, Hawaii and New Zealand for many years for export to Japan, Taiwan and Korea, it has only made an impression in the West in the last ten years. When spirulina was first introduced to the

American market in 1982, it was sold as a diet pill. Greedy entrepreneurs who had come across some Japanese research into blue-green algae seized on the fact that cyanobacteria contain chemicals which allow the brain to fool the body into thinking it is full.

Under the headline 'Doctor's Praise: A Safe Diet Pill – You'll Never Go Hungry' in *The National Enquirer*, a slimmer's miracle cure appeared to manifest. Dieters lined up outside health-food stores across the US as hundreds of spirulina-based products appeared on the shelves.

However, in the early 1980s, the entire world supply of spirulina came from Mexico and Thailand, who had long exported the bulk of their product to Japan and the Far East. Having created such an extraordinary demand for spirulina in the US – a boom that was also stimulating interest in Europe – the entrepreneurs desperately tried to eke out the small amount of spirulina available by adding bulking agents and alfalfa powder and creating increasingly low-grade products.

Soon, they faced a double dilemma: dieters were losing interest because they could not get hold of spirulina and, when they did, found that it had very little effect on their weight. What the manufacturers had failed to stress was that even high-grade blue-green algae could only help dieters as part of a controlled diet.

The boom was short-lived. Within months, word had spread and spirulina had been banished to the ranks of other 'miracle cures'. Not surprisingly, spirulina acquired a bad reputation as a health food in the US and Europe and is only beginning to be rehabilitated now that nutritionists have begun to understand its remarkable nutritional content.

The scientific community has also helped to bring spirulina back into the public eye. The Japanese Institute for Micro-algae in Tokyo has carried out some ground-breaking research into spirulina, which has been taken up by scientists in Europe and the US. (This is examined in more detail in Chapter 4.)

Spirulina is a simple one-celled microalgae which thrives in warm, alkaline water and sea water. It takes its name from the Latin word for tiny spiral, which well describes the swirling strands of the organism as they are seen under a microscope. There are thirty-five different species of spirulina growing naturally in alkaline lakes around the world – including Mexico, Kenya, Bolivia, China, Ecuador, Fiji, Indonesia, Mongolia, Japan and Burma. Some countries, most notably the US, New Zealand and Thailand, farm spirulina in vast tanks of mineral water resembling lake where conditions can be controlled so that the crops are not contaminated by other organisms or heavy metals.

In Hawaii, sea water is used as a nutrient and fed into ponds from a pipe system that reaches 2000 feet out into the ocean and to a similar depth, where the water is particularly rich in nutrients. Pure mountain water is also added, to make up for the water lost through evaporation under the sun. The ponds are harvested regularly, with 20 per cent of the spirulina recycled back into the ponds.

Much of the spirulina that reaches the shops is cultivated in farms such as those described above. However, with the recent emergence of a new blue-green algae, AFA, there has been a lot of debate about whether cultivated blue-green algae is as good as wild algae. As we shall see later on, the important distinction between the two blue-green algae is not how it grows, but the effects it has on the body or the mind/spirit. It is also a matter of taste. Some people prefer the more gentle taste of spirulina to the rather pungent taste of AFA.

It is true that cultured algae has some advantages. In the same way that farmers have developed and bred different strains of fruits and vegetables, selecting the hardiest, largest and most nutritious varieties, acquaculturists have been able to select and develop superior strains of micro-algae. Cultivated ponds are also much easier to monitor for possible toxins than natural bodies of water such as lakes or rivers, as water can be regularly checked and easily altered if there is contamination. Cultivators can also recreate ideal growing conditions all year round, ensuring that the algae grows faster and more prolifically than it ever could in the wild. Cultured spirulina grows extremely fast: typical annual production in Hawaii, for example, is more than 200,000 pounds per year.

AFA

AFA is a freshwater, wild algae which grows mainly in the northern hemisphere. Currently, the world's biggest source of AFA is Lake Klamath in southern Oregon, US, which at 140 square miles is one of the largest freshwater lakes in the world. Lake Klamath nestles among the Cascade mountains in the heart of a national park which is the major habitat of the American bald-headed eagle. As well as being ecologically protected by law, the park is also situated many miles away from industry or towns, ensuring that it is not exposed to pollution and that the environment is exceptionally pure.

Lake Klamath is also highly favoured in terms of physical geography. Since the retreat of the glaciers in the last ice age, the lake has acted as a trap for the rich supply of minerals deposited by glaciers. Moreover, seventeen rivers – called the Rivers of Light by locals because they are so pure – flow through the surrounding 4000 miles of volcanic terrain, depositing 50,000 tons of mineral-rich silt and 650 billion gallons of fresh water into the lake. Scientists estimate that nearby Mount Mazama erupted 7000 years ago, blowing off the top 5000 feet of the mountain and depositing around 35 feet of rich sediment in the area. Just one inch of the sediment is thought to support the annual algal bloom for sixty years.

Darryl Kollman, founder of US company Celltech, who first discovered Lake Klamath's AFA bloom in the late 1980s, is even more optimistic about the lake's potential role. He says: 'There is enough algae in this lake to feed all five billion inhabitants of the Earth one gram a day for the next thousand years.'

AFA blooms for just three months of the year – June, July and September – when the heat is at its most intense. Although Lake Klamath records an average 300 days of sunshine each year, the algae does not bloom during the winter months because the water temperature is too low. Although this means that less algae can be harvested, the cold mountain streams ensure that any competing bacterial growth or toxins are killed off, maintaining a pure environment for the AFA when it next comes into season.

Like spirulina, AFA is a true cyanobacterium. It collects on the surfaces of lakes in dense filaments that resemble thin blades of grass. Although some strains of AFA have produced neurotoxins (see A Note on Toxicity at the end of this chapter) in certain environmental conditions (temperature, age of culture, light intensity and acid/alkaline balance in the water), Lake Klamath AFA has never been found to be toxic and the natural environment mitigates against harmful bacteria in the water.

Many people, including doctors and scientists as we shall see later, believe that Lake Klamath blue-green algae is particularly effective in restoring the mind/spirit balance. Some believe that this is because AFA grows in the shade of Mount Shasta, which has long been regarded as a centre of extraordinary energy and spiritual power. Of course, this is impossible to prove, but it is none the less an interesting story.

Both spirulina and AFA are sold in powder, tablet, capsule and liquid forms. Again, the different forms are a matter of personal preference. Some people find the liquid and powder unappetizing and prefer tablet or capsule form; others add liquid and powder to drinks or food.

After it is harvested, blue-green algae is subjected to a variety of different treatments, including spray-drying, flash-drying, heat treatment and freezing. A great deal of research has gone into these treatments because it is important to preserve as many of the natural nutrients as possible.

Freeze-drying was popular at first because scientists discovered that heat destroys many of the algae's vital enzymes. Freeze-drying also ensures that the powder disperses easily in water, thereby making it easy to take in drinks. However, the long exposure to oxygen in this method can adversely affect its nutrient content, so spray drying has become more popular in recent years. One immediate benefit is that the algae is dried almost immediately after harvesting, ensuring that as many nutrients as possible are retained, although some heat is used.

Nutritional profile

	AFA	Spirulina
General composition		
(per cent dry organic weight)		
Protein	59%	65%
Carbohydrates	18%	18%
Lipids	4%	5%
Minerals	14%	7%
Pigments (beta carotene, chlorophyll, xanthophyll, phycocyanin, phycoerithrin)	4%	3%
Moisture	1%	2%
Essential amino acids		
(per gram)		
Isoleucine	29mg	35mg
Leucine	52mg	54mg
Lysine	35mg	29mg
Methionine	7mg	14mg
Phenylalanine	25mg	28mg
Threonine	33mg	32mg
Tryptophan	7mg	9mg
Valine	32mg	40mg
Arginine	38mg	–
Histidine	9mg	–
Non-essential amino acids		
(per gram)		
Asparagine	47mg	–
Alanine	47mg	47mg

Glutamine	78mg	91mg
Cystine	2mg	6mg
Glycine	29mg	32mg
Proline	29mg	27mg
Serine	29mg	32mg
Tyrosine	17mg	30mg
Aspartic acid	7mg	61mg
Glutamic acid	4mg	–

Mineral content
(per gram)

Boron	10.0mg	–
Calcium	14.0mg	10mg
Chlorine	464.0mcg	–
Chromium	0.5mcg	2.8mcg
Cobalt	2.0mcg	–
Copper	4.0mcg	1.2mcg
Fluorine	38.0mcg	–
Germanium	0.3mcg	0.6mcg
Iodine	0.5mcg	–
Iron	350.7mcg	1.5mg
Magnesium	2.2mg	4.0mg
Manganese	32.0mcg	50mcg
Molybdenum	3.3mcg	–
Nickel	5.3mcg	–
Phosphorus	5.1mg	9.0mg
Potassium	12.0mg	16.0mg
Selenium	0.7mcg	0.2mcg
Silicon	186.7mcg	–
Sodium	2.7mg	6.0mg
Tin	0.5mcg	–
Titanium	23.3mcg	–
Vanadium	2.7mcg	–

Zinc	18.7mcg	30.0mcg

Vitamin composition
(per gram)

Provitamin A (beta carotene)	240.0RE	230.0RE
Thiamin (B1)	4.8mcg	3.1mcg
Riboflavin (B2)	57.3mcg	35.0mcg
Pyridoxine (B6)	11.1mcg	8.0mcg
Analogue cobalamin (B12)	8.0mcg	3.2mcg
Ascorbic acid (C)	0.7mcg	–
Niacin	0.1mcg	0.1mcg
Folic acid	1.0mcg	1.0mcg
Pantothenic acid	6.8mcg	1.0mcg
Biotin	0.3mcg	0.5mcg
Vitamin E	0.1IU	0.1IU
Choline	2.3mcg	–

Fatty acid composition
(per cent lipid weight)

Palmitic (16:0)	43.4%	45.0%
Palmitoleic (16:1)	9.7%	5.6%
Palmitolinoleic (16:2)	trace	trace
Stearic (18:0)	2.9%	1.4%
Oleic (18:1)	5.0%	2.2%
Linoleic (18:2)	12.4%	17.9%
Linolenic 6, 9, 12 (18:3)	21.4%	24.9%
Cholesterol	zero	zero

Amino acids

Blue–green algae contains the following essential amino acids: lysine; tryptophan; phenylalanine; methionine; threonine; leucine; isoleucine; valine. And the following non–essential amino acids: alanine; arginine; tyrosine; glycine; glutamic acid; asparagine; histidine; serine; proline; aspartic acid.

Amino acids – or neuropeptides – help to repair, rebuild and strengthen the neurotransmitters in the brain so that the brain's neurons, or nerve cells, can communicate at 100 per cent effectiveness to the rest of the body. One of the main factors in allowing disease to gain a foothold in the body is poor electronic signals going to the brain and back to the organs and other parts of the body. In order to correct any communication problems, it is necessary to re-establish the quality of the nerve impulses so that they flow freely in both directions.

When this happens, the body comes into the natural harmony that nature intended. Lack of certain nutrients to the brain can cause severe mental and emotional imbalances as well as irritability, depression, loss of memory, lack of energy and lack of concentration (essential amino acids and B vitamins are regarded by scientists as vital for the brain to function at optimum levels).

Amino acids are the building blocks of proteins, which we need to maintain muscles and vital organs in optimum condition. Blue-green algae's proteins are biologically complete, that is to say, they provide all eight essential amino acids in the proper ratios. Most plant foods are not complete proteins because they usually lack one or more amino acids and, unfortunately, the body cannot store amino acids in anticipation of deficiencies. To synthesize protein for the body's repair and maintenance, all dietary protein factors must be present simultaneously or all the amino acids will be wasted. Even if all the complete protein is consumed, digestive difficulties can prevent assimilation of all needed elements. Blue-green algae provides all the required amino acids in a form that is five times easier to digest than meat or soya protein.

Blue-green algae contains proteins consisting of amino

acids which are hooked together in molecular chains (polypeptides). It also contain lower-weight molecular weight proteins than mature plants and other sources of protein. Some of these protein units are so small that they can be absorbed directly into the blood, where they can promote cell metabolism and help in the detoxification of harmful substances, such as cadmium and other heavy metals, nicotine and chemical toxins.

For vegetarians, or those who want to eat less meat, blue-green algae is an excellent way to maintain protein levels in the body.

Also, it is far safer to take a wholefood that contains all the essential and non-essential amino acids than to take a single, isolated amino acid. Amino acids build necessary neuropeptides which feed the delicate neurotransmitters of the brain and nervous system.

ESSENTIAL AMINO ACIDS

- **Isoleucine** is required for optimal growth, development of intelligence and maintaining the correct nitrogen equilibrium in the body. It is also used to synthesize other non-essential amino acids.
- **Leucine** stimulates brain function and increases energy levels in muscles.
- **Lysine** is the building-block of blood antibodies, strengthens the circulatory system and maintains the normal growth rate of cells. It is needed for growth, tissue repair and the production of antibodies, hormones and enzymes.

  Current research efforts are being focused on lysine's possible role in reducing the incidence of herpes infection and migraine headaches. Natural lysine deficiencies result in tiredness, inability to concentrate, irritability, bloodshot eyes, retarded growth, hair loss, anaemia and reproductive problems.

- **Methionine** is a vital lipotropic (fat- and lipid-metabolizing) amino acid that maintains the health of the liver. It is also an anti-stress factor, and can calm the nerves.
- **Phenylalanine** is required by the thyroid gland for the production of thyroxin, which stimulates the metabolic rate. Medical researchers are currently studying the role of this nutrient in overcoming depression, improving memory, increasing mental alertness, controlling allergies and as an aid to weight loss.

  Phenylalanine is one of the few amino acids which is readily converted into brain compounds that control mood. It is also needed to build proteins such as insulin, papain, melanin, and to produce adrenaline.
- **Threonine** improves intestinal function and digestive assimilation.
- **Tryptophane** increases the uptake of B vitamins, improves nerve health and the stability of emotions. Promotes a sense of calm, helps people sleep better and alleviates depression.
- **Valine** stimulates mental capacity and muscle co-ordination.

NON-ESSENTIAL AMINO ACIDS

- **Alanine** strengthens cellular walls.
- **Arginine** is important for male sexual health as seminal fluid is 80 per cent arginine. It also helps to detoxify the blood.
- **Aspartic acid** assists in the metabolism of carbohydrates into cellular energy.

- **Cystine** aids pancreatic health which stabilizes blood sugar and carbohydrate metabolism. Cystine has also been used to alleviate some symptoms of food allergy and intolerance. It builds proteins in the hair and helps destroy harmful chemicals in the body, such as acetaldehyde and free radicals produced by smoking and drinking. Cystine is also useful for preventing hangovers and preventing damage such as emphysema and lung cancer.

  It is also necessary for optimum utilization of vitamin B6, which can help against most chronic degenerative diseases, including cancer and MS.

- **Glutamic acid (glutamine)** is, with glucose, one of the principal fuels for brain cells. Has been used to reduce cravings for alcohol and to stabilize mental health. Improves intelligence, speeds the healing of ulcers, gives a lift from fatigue and helps control alcoholism, schizophrenia and cravings for sugar.

- **Glycine** promotes energy and oxygen use in cells.

- **Histidine** strengthens the nerve relays, especially in the auditory organs, and has been used to reverse some cases of deafness.

- **Proline** is a precursor of glutamic acid.

- **Serine** helps form the protective fatty sheaths surrounding nerve fibres.

- **Tyrosine** slows the ageing of cells and suppresses hunger centres in the hypothalamus. It can be synthesized from phenylalanine. Tyrosine is also involved in the proper coloration of the hair and skin and gives protection against sunburn.

  Recent clinical research has discovered that tyrosine is helpful in overcoming depression, improving memory and increasing mental alertness. Of particular interest is research linking tyrosine deficiency to the development of depression in some oral contraceptive users.

The body needs tyrosine to build many complex structural proteins and enzymes but research has centred on simpler compounds – neurotransmitters – used by the body to transmit nerve impulses and to determine mood and mental alertness. Neurotransmitters are readily formed in the body by a minor alteration of the tyrosine molecule. It is possible that deficiencies in tyrosine can impair the body's ability to produce a proper balance of neurotransmitters.

MINERALS

Blue-green algae contain all known minerals and trace elements, which are vital for the proper functioning of the body. They include: carbon; oxygen; hydrogen; nitrogen; phosphorus; sulphur; chlorine; potassium; sodium; calcium; magnesium; iron; copper; boron; manganese; zinc; silicon; cobalt; iodine; fluorine; strontium; molybdenum; bromine; vanadium; titanium; aluminium; and gallium. The most important are examined below.

- **Calcium** is the most abundant mineral in the body and is especially important for bone and dental health. It is also involved in the neural transmissions to the muscles. Calcium builds and maintains bones and teeth, helps blood to clot, aids vitality and endurance and regulates heart rhythm. It also acts to transmit nerve pulses and helps with muscle concentration.
- **Cobalt** stimulates the production of red blood cells and is the component of vitamin B12 necessary for normal growth and appetite.
- **Copper** is necessary for the absorption and utilization of

iron, which is vital for the formation of red blood cells.

- **Iron** promotes the formation of haemoglobin, the oxygen-carrying blood pigment found in healthy red blood cells. Iron deficiency is the most common mineral deficiency in the Western world, particularly among women in their reproductive years.

- **Magnesium** is necessary for calcium and vitamin C metabolism. It is essential for the normal functioning of the nervous and muscular systems. Magnesium is involved in the formation of new cells, muscle contraction and nerve functions, assists with energy production and forms part of the mineral structure of bones. It also helps the assimilation of vitamin C, B vitamins and protein. Magnesium deficiency can lead to spasmodic muscle disorders, including cardiac irregularities.

- **Manganese** activates enzyme systems, along with zinc, and other minerals. Its activity is related to the proper utilization of vitamins B1 and E. Manganese promotes the activity of neurotransmitter acetylcholine, and helps stabilize blood sugar.

- **Phosphorous** is the second most abundant material in the human body – it is found in practically every cell. It functions with calcium to maintain bone and teeth density and helps digest carbohydrates, calcium, vitamin D and B vitamins niacin and riboflavin.

- **Potassium** is a crucial mineral that regulates the body's electrolyte balance. Potassium deficiency can cause heart arrest, hypertension, adrenal exhaustion and muscular collapse. It also works with sodium to control fluid balance and muscle and nerve functions and is vital for muscle tone, nerves, heart action and enzyme reactions.

- **Selenium** was originally thought to be a toxic heavy metal, but is now known to be necessary for health. It

slows down ageing, harmful oxidation and free-radical
formation, reduces the toxic effect of carcinogens and
improves cardiac efficiency.

- **Sodium** helps to control body fluid balance and is
involved in muscle and nerve functions.
- **Zinc** is the pivot for more than thirty vital enzymatic
reactions and has a profound effect on mental health, skin
tone, prostate function and healing capacity. Zinc helps
normal tissue function, and protein, carbohydrate and fat
metabolism. It also helps to heal wounds, assists the
immune system and is necessary for building cells.

Vitamins

Blue-green algae contains the following vitamins, which are
necessary to carry on the metabolic process: vitamin A; vitamin
C; vitamin E; vitamins B12, B1 and B2; nicotinic acid/niacin;
folic acid; pantothenic acid; vitamin B6; biotin and inositol.

- **Vitamin A** builds resistance to infections, especially of the
respiratory tract. It also helps maintain a healthy condition
of the outer layers of many tissues and organs and promotes
healthy growth and vitality. Vitamin A is essential for
normal colour vision and for the red cells in the eye that
enable us to see in dim light. It promotes healthy skin and
mucous membranes lining the mouth, nose and digestive
system and permits the formation of visual purple in the
eye, counteracting night blindness and weak eyesight. It is
also essential for lactating and pregnant women.
- **Vitamin B (pantothenic acid)** is the 'stress' vitamin
which is used by the adrenal glands, along with cholesterol
and vitamin C, to manufacture cortisone and other steroids
in response to physical and mental stress. Like vitamin A, it

promotes healthy hair, skin and growth and helps
manufacture antibodies to fight infection, and also
metabolizes food for energy. Deficiency of pantothenic
acid encourages sensitivity to allergy, infection, and
degenerative diseases such as arthritis and rheumatism.
Ulcers and hypoglycaemia have also been associated with a
shortage of this vitamin.

- **Cyanobalamin (B12)** is the most difficult of all vitamins
  to obtain from vegetable sources. Blue-green algae is
  extremely rich in this rare vitamin and is thought to
  contain 250 per cent more than beef liver, previously
  thought to be nature's richest source. B12 deficiency
  results in pernicious anaemia, nerve degeneration,
  premature senility, pronounced fatigue and mental illness
  resembling schizophrenia.

  B12 is also needed for normal nerve function and for
  red blood cell manufacture, helping protect against
  anaemia. It is used for protein, fat and carbohydrate
  metabolism. It also promotes growth and increased
  appetite in children and is a general tonic for adults.

- **Pyridoxine (B6)** is involved in the breakdown and
  assimilation of protein, fat and carbohydrates. It promotes
  normal blood cell formation, protects cardiac health,
  reduces oedema and stabilizes female hormone levels.
  Pyridoxine prevents various nervous and skin disorders and
  nausea. Together with zinc, it has been shown to cure
  some forms of schizophrenia. High doses can also help to
  alleviate symptoms of PMS.

- **Riboflavin/B2**. The most common vitamin deficiency is
  that of riboflavin, which results in cataracts, failing vision,
  watery eyes and uncontrollable eczema. B2 improves
  growth, promotes general health and is essential for
  healthy eyes, skin and mouth.

- **Thiamin/B1** is a co-enzyme in the breakdown of dietary carbohydrate. It maintains levels of glucose in the blood. Deficiency results in weakness, cardiac damage, abdominal distension and poor oxygenation. Severe shortages result in death, as critical toxaemia develops from unmetabolized carbohydrate fragments. Thiamin promotes growth, aids digestion and is essential for the normal functioning of nerve tissues, muscles and heart.

- **Biotin** is an enzyme that carries carbon dioxide during certain biochemical reactions involved in carbohydrate metabolism. It also acts as a co-enzyme in the assimilation of other B-complex vitamins. Biotin is destroyed by eating raw egg whites and some kinds of fish. It is also involved in manufacture of fatty acids and glycogen and in protein metabolism needed for normal growth/development.

- **Vitamin C/ascorbic acid** is necessary for healthy teeth, gums and bones. It strengthens all connective tissue, promotes wound healing and is very important for maintaining general health. Vitamin C is vital for the growth and repair of body cells; it helps form collagen in connective tissue; promotes healthy blood vessels, gums and teeth; produces haemoglobin and red blood cells; manufactures adrenalin; and is an extremely powerful antioxidant.

- **Vitamin D** controls the absorption of calcium from the intestine and helps to regulate the metabolism of calcium. It prevents rickets developing in children and osteomalacia in adults by helping to regulate bone formation.

- **Tocopherol/vitamin E** Blue-green algae contains more vitamin E gram per gram than pure wheatgerm, one of the richest sources of the vitamin. Tocopherol protects heart and vascular health, promotes the oxygenation of cells and retards ageing. As an antioxidant, it protects tissues against free-radical damage and promotes normal growth and development. It also helps normal blood cell production.

- **Folic acid** is essential to proper haemoglobin formation in red blood cells. Deficiency of folic acid results in anaemia, poor growth, skin pigmentation disorders and premature greying of the hair. It is essential in the formation of DNA and necessary for red blood cell manufacture.

- **Inositol** is a vital nutrient that sustains liver health and helps detoxify carcinogens, particularly excess female hormones. It also helps normalize blood cholesterol levels. With choline, inositol is used by the liver to manufacture lecithin. Inositol is the second most abundant vitamin in the body after niacin.

  Recent studies have shown that inositol, with biotin, reduces loss of scalp hair.

- **Niacin** is also known as nicotinic acid and niacinamide, which is an alternative form. Niacin is essential to mental health. Some doctors, most notably Dr Abram Hoffer, a pioneer of orthomolecular psychiatry in the US, has completely relieved schizophrenia symptoms in some patients by using niacin in his treatment regimes. Niacin is also regarded as an effective agent to lower cholesterol.

Natural pigments

While the protein, mineral and vitamin content of blue-green algae is impressive, it is also rich in the enzymatic pigments that are biochemically important to life. Without these pigments, organisms could not synthesize many of the enzymes necessary for balancing metabolism.

The two most important pigments in blue-green algae are phycocyanin, which gives it its distinctive blue tinge, and chlorophyll, which lends the green colour. In addition, it contains the following pigments: phycobilins; phycobiliproteins; phycoerithrin; xanthophyll; xhrysolaminarin; beta carotene (see below); flavacene; myxoxanthin; oscilloxanthin; fucoxanthin; myxoxanthophyll; other carotenoids; and allophycocyanin.

CHLOROPHYLL

The most visible pigment in algae is chlorophyll, a green molecule common to all plants. Chlorophyll releases ions when struck by the energy of sunlight. These ions then proceed to stimulate the biochemical reactions that form proteins, vitamins and sugars. Chlorophyll has been called 'plant blood' as it has a very similar make-up to haemoglobin, the oxygen-carrying red pigment in our own blood. Both are constructed of almost identical molecular structures, called pyrrole rings, and both substances are called 'porphyrin pigments' by scientists.

The only difference between blood and chlorophyll is that chlorophyll has a magnesium ion at its core, while blood has iron in the centre of the molecule. Magnesium imparts the green colour to the chlorophyll molecule and is involved in the synthesis of other materials, whereas iron gives haemoglobin a red colour and changes the function of the porphyrin molecule to enable respiration and the breakdown of foodstuffs and other chemicals.

In photosynthesis, plants use chlorophyll and sunlight to convert water and carbon dioxide from the air into sugar. Some scientists are of the opinion that if chlorophyll is ingested with sufficient iron, its magnesium ion can be displaced to yield a haemoglobin molecule.

Experiments in Japan have demonstrated that blue-green algae has a marked positive effect on anaemia, possibly due to the conversion of chlorophyll into haemoglobin. Chlorophyll is absorbed directly through the cell membranes in the mouth, throat, stomach and intestines and is an excellent blood purifier.

PHYCOCYANIN AND OTHERS

The pigment which gives algae its blue cast is phycocyanin, which is related to the human pigment bilirubin, important for healthy liver function and digestion of amino acids. Another important pigment is porphyrin, a red compound that forms the active nucleus of haemoglobin. Related to this structure is the polypyrrole molecule of B12 which is essential to the formation of healthy red blood cells. These and lesser pigments such as phycoerythrin, tetrapyrrole and phytonadione and the carotenoids are not just the colour of living organisms; they are used to carry on metabolic processes throughout the body. Without them, enzymatic reactions would be reduced until cellular disintegration occurred.

Enzymes

There are literally thousands of enzymes in algae. Enzymes, along with their co-factors (co-enzymes), vitamins and minerals, do all the work of the body, including prevention of disease and healing. Certain enzymes break down or metabolize proteins, fats, carbohydrates, fibre and anything composed of these substances. This includes circulating immune complexes (CICs), which are produced by the antigens and antibodies found in areas of the body where there is inflammation. Enzymes depolymerize, or break up, these CICs, thereby aiding the healing process.

Essential fatty acids

It is hard to imagine that a concentrated source of vitamins such as blue-green algae is not also loaded with fats, starches and calories. Yet blue-green algae has only a 7 per cent lipid (fat) content, most of which is in the form of essential fatty acids, which help to normalize and lower cholesterol levels in the blood.

The essential fatty acids are sometimes called vitamin F and include linoleic, linolenic and arachidonic acid. They are used by the body to manufacture prostaglandins, the hormone regulators of blood pressure and capillary resistance. They are also involved in respiration in cells and are especially important for transporting oxygen. They affect the health of the hair, skin and nails and help break up cholesterol in the bloodstream.

Unlike many fats, essential fatty acids are not dangerous, but are absolutely vital to health. These provide the most concentrated sources of energy for the body; they function as carriers for vitamins A, D, E and K and are important in the conversion of plant beta carotene into vitamin A. Algae contains very little starch or sugar. What carbohydrate it does supply, roughly 10–15 per cent, is primarily in the form of polysaccharides, rhamnose and glycogen. These two polysaccharides are easily absorbed by human cells with minimum intervention by insulin, thus placing no strain on the pancreas. Hence they provide speedy energy without taxing the pancreas or precipitating hypoglycaemia.

The lipids found in blue-green algae are commonly known as glycolipids, meaning that they are composed of a sugar portion and a lipid portion. They also function to provide the body with a uniform level of energy, not the up-and-down energy cycle of the kind that results from refined white sugar (hypoglycaemia).

As far as calories are concerned, algae is also very good: there are only 3.9 calories per gram, compared with 65 calories per gram of beef.

It is a mistake to believe that you can get all your essential fatty acids from processed vegetable oils because the oil becomes degraded during processing.

Essential fatty acids are important in all immune processes and are another substance on the list required for healthy skin. Gamma linoleic acid (GLA), which is protectively embedded in food but readily available for use, is very important as a precursor to prostaglandin PGE1, which is a vasodilator, inhibits thrombosis and the proliferation of cancer cells, helps control blood pressure and regulate brain function, and is involved in the burning of fat, an important factor in weight control and energy production.

Carotenoids

Plant foods contain certain substances which are not true vitamins, but are precursors from which the body can then synthesize the appropriate vitamins. The carotenoid compounds of blue-green algae are used to produce vitamin A. True vitamin A in its preformed state is found only in animal sources such as liver. However, this form of vitamin A is sometimes associated with toxicity, since it is fat-soluble and is not easily excreted from the body.

In contrast, carotenoid complexes found in vegetable foods are converted into vitamin A only as and when they are needed, thus minimizing the dangers of toxic build-up. Blue-green algae is a primary source of vitamin A precursors – scientists and nutritionists believe that fish derive and concentrate vitamin A in their livers from the vast quantities of algae they consume. Algae also contains the yellow/orange pigment, cryptoxanthine and beta carotene from which vitamin A can be made.

A note on toxicity

It is true that industry standards have not yet been fully adopted to ensure the quality of blue-green algae, but most of the big producers, such as AquaSource, Celltech, Earthrise and Nature's Choice are responsible companies which employ their own scientists to check for toxins and ensure high levels of quality control. An indication of blue-green algae's safety is that it has never been banned by the ultra-cautious US Food and Drugs Administration (FDA), which will clamp down immediately on any product which is thought to be dangerous to the public.

Yet, in recent years, there has been much speculation about whether blue-green algae can harbour dangerous toxins. Much of this stemmed from a paper published in the *Scientific American* (January, 1994) by Wayne W. Carmichael, professor of aquatic biology and toxicology at Wright State University. Entitled 'The Toxins of Cyanobacteria', it included AFA among the toxic algae cited. Pharmaceutical companies and health-food stores in the US over-reacted, claiming that AFA was poisonous, but failed to indicate that the reference to toxic AFA was a single strain at a single site in the north-east US, not at Lake Klamath, where all the AFA for the health-food market is produced.

The article actually said that no other reports of that strain had been observed or recorded and must therefore be considered anomalous. This is backed up by an article in the *Journal of Applied Phycology* (1993), which stated that AFA found in Lake Klamath was not capable of producing toxins.

The truth of the matter is that very few of the estimated 1500 species of blue-green algae are known to be toxic. A survey of world scientific research on cyanobacteria indicates that there are only two poisonous species: *Anabaena flos-aquae* and *Microcystis aeruginosa*, both of which can produce toxins that can be dangerous to animals, including human beings. But it must be noted that these two strains do not produce toxins all the time, nor do all strains of these two species produce toxins.

According to some sources, confusion over the toxicity of blue-green algae stems from inaccurate historical reports from the last century, when biologists were just starting to understand the biological and chemical impact of algae on bodies of water. They often described algal growth as a bloom which suffocated drainage, killed the lake, destroyed waters and was deadly to canals. What they meant was that the algal bloom cut off light, causing other plants in the water to die, which meant that animals dependent on the water and plants for their survival also died. By a quirk of semantics, the notion of death was inextricably tied up with algae, whether or not it was itself toxic.

There was also confusion over the names *Anabaena flos-aquae* and *Aphanizomenon flos-aquae* (AFA). One science writer in the last century confused AFA with *Anabaena flos-aquae* and, despite many attempts to change this, the toxic label unfortunately stuck to AFA.

Although it is true to say that infinitesimal traces of toxins have been found in Lake Klamath AFA, there have been no reported intoxications in the area of fish, wildlife or humans. Research by Dr Larry Barton at the University of New Mexico has not indicated toxicity whatsoever in mice injected with Klamath Lake algae.

Lake Klamath AFA has been consumed by thousands of people around the world without any negative effects being reported. Scientists think that this may be for a number of reasons:

- the strains growing at Lake Klamath may not be capable of producing a toxin;
- the chemical and physical factors (certain combinations of light and heat) for toxins to survive are not present and therefore toxin production is not stimulated;
- some type of biological or physical factor may cause the rapid degeneration of the toxin when it is formed, perhaps because the lake is highly alkaline; or
- the toxin is destroyed during processing.

Some people have complained of minor allergenic reactions to blue-green algae and there are a few cases of skin irritation in people who have swum in water densely populated with AFA. Yet AFA has been handled daily by hundreds of people during harvesting and production, and none has reportedly complained of allergies on their hands, faces or arms.

Most manufacturers advise anyone who is worried about traces of toxins in AFA to consider the fact that many fruits and vegetables also contain substances which can be toxic in a very pure form. These include caffeine in coffee and chocolate and solanine in potatoes, both of which are potentially lethal. However, these foods rarely – if ever – cause illness or death. Indeed, it is almost impossible to think of a food that would not cause some allergic reaction in at least one person in the world. Many species of mushroom are poisonous, but most people eat them. The important thing to remember about AFA is that its toxicity is constantly monitored throughout all stages of harvesting and production to ensure that it is safe for human consumption. In fact, blue-green algae has probably been more thoroughly investigated than the majority of foods animals and humans consume.

Chapter 4

THE BLUE-GREEN HEALER

Blue-green algae's second revolution

Each one of the substances of a man's diet acts upon his body and changes it in some way and upon these changes his whole life depends, whether he be in health, in sickness, or in convalescence.

Hippocrates

Blue-green algae is the focus of extensive medical research across the world at present because of its remarkable detoxifying powers. The applications for this are obvious: AIDS, cancer, degenerative disorders, such as arthritis and ME, and radiation sickness. Much of this research has been spurred on by the remarkable anecdotal evidence for blue-green algae's regenerative powers – like many plants and herbs, blue-green algae has a long history of use as a powerful healing agent. Now, the scientific and medical community have finally woken up to its potential.

To date, most of the scientific and clinical research into the effects of blue-green algae on human health have been carried out using spirulina. However, AFA shares a remarkably similar nutritional profile and many scientists believe it has comparable health-giving properties, and the added benefit of being able to rebalance the left–right brain function (this is discussed more fully in Chapter 7).

Although several feeding trials on animals, including rats,

chickens and pigs, have been carried out in the US, most of the studies on the effects of blue-green algae on humans have been carried out in Mexico (a large production centre for spirulina) and Japan (the world's largest consumer of blue-green algae and Mexico's biggest export market). The majority of these studies conclude that blue-green algae is a useful adjunct to any therapeutic programme, especially those where the root cause of the illness is chronic malnutrition.

Most nutritionists will agree that blue-green algae's most useful role is as a preventive agent against disease. Its perfectly balanced nutrition helps the relatively healthy body to work more efficiently, enabling it to extract maximum nutrition from food, fight off infections, increase stamina and mental sharpness and speed up the body's elimination processes, thereby relieving the body of toxins which can cause fatigue and even depression. Not surprisingly, with the body functioning properly, there can be significant improvements in mood and temperament.

For people in different stages of sickness, blue-green algae is a useful supplement. For those whose food intake is limited, it is a light, but nutritious source of proteins, vitamins and minerals, and it is also a powerful detoxifier for anyone undergoing high doses of drugs or medication, such as chemotherapy.

Ultimately, blue-green algae appears to stimulate the body's cellular memory or genetic code (DNA), which in turn appears to stimulate the formation of new cells, assisting the healing process.

In this chapter, we shall look at some of the conditions blue-green algae has been shown to be effective against and look at the overall beneficial effects it has on healthy people.

A–Z of healthy effects

AIDS

In 1989, the US National Cancer Institute announced that chemicals extracted from cyanobacteria had shown to be extremely effective in laboratory tests against the HIV virus. Much of the research focused on blue-green algae's sulpholipids which were part of its glycolipid content. Both spirulina and AFA contain glycolipids and sulpholipids. A larger testing programme, using animals, is now under way.

In April 1996, there was an even more dramatic break-through when scientists from the Laboratory of Viral Pathogenesis, the Dana Faber Cancer Institute, Harvard Medical School and Earthrise Farms in California announced: 'Water extract of spirulina platensis inhibits HIV-1 replication in human-derived T-cells and in human mononuclear cells. A concentration of 5–10mg/ml was found to reduce viral production.'

In simple terms, the announcement said that five–ten grams of spirulina halted the HIV virus in laboratory tests. Higher concentrations of spirulina, meanwhile, prevented the virus replicating itself – effectively stopping it. Significantly, the scientists reported that even extremely high doses of spirulina were not toxic to human cells.

On the other side of the world, in Japan, a group of medical students published a study last year on Calcium-Spirulan, a spirulina extract which has also been shown to inhibit the HIV virus. The researchers discovered that Calcium-Spirulan inhibits the replication of HIV-1, Herpes Simplex, Human Cytomegalovirus, Influenza-A virus and both the mumps and measles viruses in laboratory tests, yet was also found to be very safe for human cells.

The scientists explained that Calcium-Spirulan is a poly-merized sugar molecule, containing both calcium and sulphur, which acts as a barrier membrane to the human cell, thereby preventing the virus from penetrating the cell and infecting it. The virus remains stuck outside the cell barrier, unable to replicate itself, and the body eventually eliminates it.

Obviously, these two breakthroughs are of great importance to both the medical community and anyone suffering from AIDS or is HIV-positive. It seems likely that a great deal of future research will be based on blue-green algae, particularly spirulina, not only for its ability to slow down the HIV virus, but also as a preventive agent against this terrible disease.

Allergies (see also Immune Disorders)

Several Japanese studies into children's food allergies have found that blue-green algae is a vital food source for infants who are allergic both to cows' milk and soya-based baby foods. Babies who were fed blue-green algae put on weight and became less susceptible to other food allergies in later life.

US researchers are currently exploring the benefits of blue-green algae in people who are particularly sensitive to seasonal pollen allergies, such as hay fever. Early results show that sensitivity to high pollen levels has decreased among people who have taken blue-green algae supplements.

Alzheimer's disease

Much of the work on blue-green algae's effects on Alzheimer's disease has been carried out by US physician Dr Gabriel Cousens. Using mainly AFA, which he discovered had many brain-enhancing qualities, including improved concentration and mental clarity, Dr Cousens found that

AFA partially reversed Alzheimer's disease in one patient and halted rapidly advancing senility in another.

Dr Cousens gave AFA to a sixty-four-year-old lawyer who had suffered with Alzheimer's disease for three years and appeared to be deteriorating rapidly. After a month, the degeneration appeared to be slowing down and he remained in a stable condition for three further years. However, when he stopped taking AFA, his condition began to worsen, but once he started taking AFA again, the degeneration slowed down.

Anaemia

Many women suffer iron deficiencies or anaemia for a large part of their lives, particularly during their reproductive years. Women need to be more careful than men in monitoring their iron levels, because they generally do not eat as much meat as men and also lose iron when they menstruate each month. Iron is the single most common mineral deficiency in the world and affects children, older people and dieters as well as women. It is absolutely vital for a healthy immune system.

In clinical tests, blue-green algae has increased the volume of red blood cells in the body, and their capacity to carry oxygen, in thirty days. Scientists think it is the high levels of iron, chlorophyll, vitamin B12, folic acid and protein which are behind blue-green algae's efficacy in treating anaemia. Blue-green algae is also particularly beneficial in treating long-term anaemia with underlying malnutrition and rapid blood-loss anaemia.

In another study, rats who were fed spirulina were found to absorb 60 per cent more iron than animals fed iron sulphate supplements, which suggests that iron in blue-green algae is more easily assimilated than iron from other sources.

A Japanese study of eight young women whose blood haemoglobin had been affected by long-term dieting were cured of anaemia in thirty days, after taking four grams of spirulina after each meal. In another Japanese study, the red blood count of anaemic animals returned to normal within four-and-a-half days of administering algae.

Some researchers believe that blue-green algae is so effective in treating anaemia because of its high chlorophyll content (often called 'plant blood'). They think that the body manages to convert chlorophyll into haemoglobin, by displacing chlorophyll's magnesium nucleus with an iron nucleus.

Arthritis

Although there have been no scientific studies into the effects of blue-green algae on arthritis specifically, there is much anecdotal evidence that it is especially beneficial in treating degenerative diseases such as this.

Scientists believe that one of the reasons for the rise in cases of arthritis and other degenerative diseases is that our diets have become extremely reliant on saturated fats which may prevent essential fatty acids from working properly in our bodies. Gamma linoleic acid (GLA) is an essential fatty acid which has an important role in many bodily functions, including the synthesis of cholesterol (see below), regulating blood pressure and managing inflammations.

Clinical studies have shown that GLA can help with symptoms of arthritis: blue-green algae has more naturally occurring GLA than any other foodstuff on Earth with the exception of one – human breast milk.

Cancer

Cancer is one of the biggest killers in the Western world. Although more and more people seem to be succumbing to cancer, we are still no closer to discovering a cure for the disease. However, we do know that diet is an important factor in the onset of the disease and that some foods can actually protect against it.

During the last twenty years, scientists have studied different foods for possible protective agents against cancer as well as highly carcinogenic foods. One breakthrough they have made is the discovery that people who eat large amounts of fruits and vegetables tend to suffer a lower incidence of cancer, particularly stomach, colon, breast and cervical cancer.

Between 1975 and 1986, fifteen studies in the US showed a correlation between high levels of beta carotene and vitamin A – which are found in many fruits and vegetables – and a lower incidence of lung cancer. One study showed that smoking increases the risks of lung cancer, not only because it contains powerful carcinogens in the smoke, but also because it destroyed beta carotene in the body.

Scientists at the Albert Einstein College of Medicine in the US have also shown that beta carotene helps protect against cervical cancer and skin cancer. Research elsewhere has shown that spirulina has successfully reversed squamous-cell skin carcinoma and destroyed pre-cancer squamous-cell carcinoma. Moreover, three-quarters of people studied who were extremely sensitive to sunlight found that they were able to remain in the sun four times longer than usual after taking spirulina.

Beta carotene's most important function, it appears, is in stimulating the immune system and destroying the rogue scavenger cells – free radicals – which can damage normal, healthy cells. Beta carotene is a powerful antioxidant, that is, it has the ability to join up with a free radical and deactivate it. When antioxidants are present in the body, the cells are no longer in danger of being damaged. Small amounts of free radicals are produced during breathing and digestion, but exposure to high levels of pollution, sunlight, smoke and bacterial infections can trigger dangerously high levels of free radicals in the body. Once they are formed, they can cause a reaction that can produce yet more free radicals in the body.

Many scientists believe that some cancers are the result of these damaged cells running amok, causing cells to grow at an uncontrolled rate. Once cells have been damaged, they lose their ability to function normally. Although researchers have developed special enzymes which can repair damaged DNA in these cells, the cells can revert to their previous state if they are exposed to toxins or radiation through smoking.

New research has found that beta carotene is of vital importance in the way our cells communicate with each other. Scientists believe that cancerous cell lines are unable to accept chemical signals from other cells which could control their growth. Beta carotene appears to open up the communication processes between normal and pre-cancerous and cancerous cells, thereby enabling the body to send signals which could stop cancerous cells dividing. In this way, beta carotene is thought to have the potential to reverse cancer.

Blue-green algae also contains high levels of caretonoids, such as cryptoxanthin and lutein, which are used by the body to produce vitamin A. Vitamin A is a very powerful protective agent against cancer and is found in its true state only in animal protein, such as liver, which means that some vegetarians are deficient in the vitamin. Too much vitamin A, however, can be toxic as it is not excreted from the body very easily.

Early research has shown that the sort of caretonoids found in blue-green algae are powerful agents in reducing the size of malignant tumours. Tumours which have been induced in hamsters in clinical trials have regressed when treated with extracts from algae.

Chemotherapy sickness

Radiotherapy and chemotherapy in the treatment of cancer can cause many unwelcome side-effects, including depressed immune systems as the therapies can kill the body's white defence cells (leucocytes). Clinical studies have shown that 2–3g of spirulina slows the loss of these cells and that patients who take it during treatment experience less nausea and fatigue.

Cholesterol levels

A Japanese study at the University of Tokai found that 4g of spirulina per day significantly improved the health of thirty men who suffered high cholesterol, mild hypertension and hyperlipidaemia. After eight weeks of taking 4g of spirulina a day, one group reported lower cholesterol levels even though they did not change their diets in any other respect. Another group, which took the spirulina for only four weeks, also found that cholesterol levels fell, although they began to creep up again soon after the group stopped taking the supplement.

The researchers concluded that blue-green algae is a useful food for controlling cholesterol levels, particularly as no side-effects were noted in either group. They also drew a comparison with the beneficial effects of dietary fish oil in reducing cholesterol. Like fish oil, blue-green algae contains high levels of gamma linoleic acid (GLA), an essential fatty acid. The researchers concluded that fish themselves derive their own GLA from micro-algae, such as plankton.

Chronic fatigue syndrome

Chronic fatigue syndrome (CFS) has been linked to many things, including poor nutrition, immune system depression, toxic overload, viral infections, and, most recently, accumulations of organophosphates. It will take many more years and studies before we know for certain what is really behind this debilitating illness, which strikes down many young people, even children as young as eight years old.

Although no clinical study has been conducted on the effects of blue-green algae on CFS, there is much anecdotal evidence that it can steadily reverse the symptoms of the disease, which include dizziness, panic attacks, chronic tiredness, muscle pain and headaches. The reason for this is that blue-green algae is both a potent detoxifier and a high quality food source. Moreover, its high levels of protein, vitamins and minerals are very easily absorbed by the body and therefore put no strain on the immune system or other bodily systems which may be under stress.

Depression

Dr Gabriel Cousens' pioneering work in the US on AFA's remarkable effects on Alzheimer's disease and its value as a pure brain food has stimulated many people to take blue-green algae in order to rectify imbalances in the brain which may cause depression. Again, although clinical studies on the subject are eagerly awaited, there is much anecdotal evidence. Many people, especially the elderly and long-term depressed, have reported a significant improvement in vitality and well-being after taking blue-green algae.

Diabetes

Japanese clinical trials have shown that when diabetic patients were given twenty-one tablets of spirulina each day, their diabetes improved within weeks and they experienced significant weight loss. The scientists also reported that patients' overall stamina, energy and well-being were improved when they took blue-green algae.

Researchers think that blue-green algae is effective in treating diabetes because it contains polysaccharide sugars which are very readily assimilated by the body and maintain a steady blood sugar level. Another advantage was that blue-green algae helped to curb food cravings because the nutrients it supplies are so comprehensive that it satisfies the body. Weight loss and reduced sugar craving meant that patients did not need as much insulin.

Digestive problems

Blue-green algae has been shown to stimulate the growth of healthy bacteria in the intestines. Research in Japan showed that spirulina increased lactobacillus in rats by 300 per cent over one hundred days, compared with a control group. Vitamin B1 absorption also improved by 43 per cent and the researchers concluded that blue-green algae increases both lactobacillus and the absorption of vitamin B1.

Healthy lactobacillus promotes bowel health by preventing constipation, fighting infections and helping to detoxify potentially poisonous chemicals in our food. As well as keeping the gut healthy and improving elimination, it helps with digestion and absorption of food and stimulates the immune system.

Healthy lactobacillus is particularly important for AIDS patients, as the inability to absorb nutrients in the intestines can cause serious immune deficiency and malnutrition. AIDS researchers have discovered that in HIV-1 patients, malabsorption of nutrients is often associated with opportunistic infections which can trigger full-blown AIDS. Doctors recommend that HIV patients take high quality nutrient and lactobacillus supplements to maintain healthy intestinal flora and prevent infection.

Fertility

Nutritionists agree that the best way to maintain and protect fertility is to eat a well-balanced diet which ensures the body has a store of vitamins to draw from, particularly in times of stress. This ensures that the endocrine system, which controls the production of hormones, is properly regulated. Moreover, studies of rats fed blue-green algae have shown that they have improved fertility, which is not surprising since it contains all the essential proteins, vitamins and minerals.

Gum disease

In 1941, an American dentist, S.L. Goldberg, successfully treated 300 patients suffering from pyorrhoea (bleeding gums and loosening teeth) with liquid chlorophyll. He discovered that those who were also suffering from Vincent's disease, a gum infection which is caused by lack of B-complex vitamins and exacerbated by stress, also improved significantly.

Dr Goldberg encouraged his patients to squirt liquid chlorophyll between their teeth at least four times a day and also to rinse their mouths with a chlorophyll-based mouthwash. Soon, he found that his patients' teeth tightened in the gums, the bleeding stopped and new tissue grew over the gums to replace damaged tissue.

Chlorophyll was used extensively on the battlefields of the First and Second World Wars as an emergency procedure to disinfect wounds, prevent infection and promote healing in damaged tissue. Blue-green algae has an extremely high chlorophyll content – in fact, it is entirely responsible for its green pigment (phycocyanin is the blue pigment). Taking blue-green algae will thus ensure rapid healing of damaged tissue, as well as providing a concentrated source of vitamin C and calcium, both of which are necessary to maintain the health of teeth and gums.

Heart disease

A ten-year study into beta carotene's effect on cancer, currently under way at Harvard Medical School, surprisingly revealed in an interim report that of 333 doctors who were showing signs of coronary heart disease at the outset of the study, those who took extra beta carotene suffered half as many heart attacks, strokes and heart surgical operations as those who did not. The researchers acknowledged that beta carotene is as useful an agent for controlling heart disease as it is for cancer.

Beta carotene also appears to prevent the formation and oxidation of low-density lipoprotein (LDL) cholesterol, thereby ensuring that the arteries do not become blocked. Blue-green algae contains extremely high levels of both 'cis' and 'trans' beta carotene.

Heavy metal poisoning

After the war, Japan's rapid drive towards industrial supremacy resulted in several environmental disasters involving heavy metals. Consequently, there have been many studies in Japan into the effects of heavy metal pollution on health. Scientists have found that blue-green algae is particularly effective in helping the body rapidly to eliminate contaminants such as cadmium, lead and mercury, with no adverse effects on patients.

Hypertension

Experiments in Japan have also shown that chlorophyll is a very powerful agent for increasing blood circulation to all the organs in the body by dilating blood vessels. In the heart itself, it appears to aid the transmission of nerve impulses that control contraction; the heart rate is slowed, yet each contraction is more powerful, improving the overall efficiency of the heart.

Blue-green algae has very high levels of chlorophyll, but low levels of sodium. Most hypertension patients are limited to 2000mg or less of sodium each day, which means that they cannot eat kelp or seaweed-based supplements, which have very high sodium contents. Freshwater algae has such tiny amounts of sodium that it is safe for those with even severe hypertension.

Immune disorders

The immune system is our first line of defence against disease, whether infectious or degenerative. Its role is to stop trouble in the body before it starts, for example destroying pre-cancerous cells before they take hold in the body. Studies on animals have shown that beta carotene can act as a powerful stimulant to the immune system.

Spirulina and AFA are both powerful tonics for the immune system, no doubt because of their high beta carotene content. Studies on mice, hamsters, chickens, cats and fish have shown that blue-green algae can significantly improve immune system function. It appears to stimulate the cellular immune system, which consists of macrophages (which kill germs), T-cells, bone marrow stem cells, B-cells and natural killer cells. These cells circulate in organs vital to the immune system – the liver, spleen, thymus, lymph nodes, adenoids, tonsils and bone marrow. Blue-green algae appears to revitalize these cells and organs, improving their ability to function in the face of stress from environmental toxins or infectious diseases.

US doctors believe that even small amounts of blue-green algae (especially spirulina) can help rejuvenate the thymus gland, the pivotal gland in the immune system, and the spleen. It also seems to be particularly effective in stimulating the pituitary and pineal glands.

Research in China has focused on the pigment phycocyanin in blue-green algae, which gives the algae its distinctive colour. Phycocyanin appears to affect the stem cells found in bone marrow, which are vitally important for the immune system. Stem cells are known as 'grandmother cells' to both white blood cells, which make up the immune system, and red blood cells, which oxygenate the body.

Chinese scientists have also found that phycocyanin can stimulate the production of red blood cells, emulating the effect of the hormone erythropoietin (EPO), which is produced by healthy kidneys and regulates the production of red blood cells by bone marrow stem cells.

Liver disease

The liver is one of the main eliminative organs in the body and needs a good source of high quality, easily assimilable protein to keep it functioning at its optimum level. When it is under assault from toxins, alcohol or infection, it needs even more nutrients to function properly.

Japanese studies on patients with severe liver disease, including acute and chronic hepatitis and cirrhosis through alcohol abuse, revealed that blue-green algae can boost the liver's effectiveness within two to six weeks.

Malnutrition

Because blue-green algae is so densely packed with nutrients, gram per gram, it is the perfect food for malnourished people – infants, children, the sick and the elderly. Both spirulina and AFA have high levels of protein which can be assimilated very easily by the body. They also contain all the essential amino acids, vitamins, minerals and trace elements, beta carotene and gamma linoleic acid that are essential for the healthy maintenance of the body.

Blue-green algae is widely recommended by nutritionists in the West for people who are severely undernourished as a result of poor diets high in refined foods, cholesterol, sugar and fat. Spirulina has been donated to many humanitarian projects around the world, including in India, Nicaragua, Togo, Brazil and Cambodia (see Chapter 9), with spectacular results.

Finally, African tribes that incorporate blue-green algae into their diet have been shown to suffer virtually no malnutrition, even when surrounding tribes have been stricken by famine. The most notable example is the Kanembu tribe of

Chad, central Africa, who have traditionally eaten blue-green algae harvested from Lake Chad.

Pancreatitis

The pancreas regulates blood sugar levels and the synthesis of digestive enzymes. The pancreas can become stressed when the body is subjected to a poor diet and excess alcohol and sugar. After a while, the gland begins to malfunction and fails to send enzymes into the stomach and intestines to process food. These enzymes instead attack the tissues in the pancreas, causing swelling in the abdomen, and blood sugars go out of control, causing sugar cravings and food intolerances. The body, meanwhile, fails to absorb nutrients and proteins, which can lead to malnutrition and, ultimately, serious disease.

Blue-green algae is used extensively in Japan for people who suffer pancreatitis because its natural enzymes and balanced nutrition can reverse the symptoms of the condition.

Pre-menstrual syndrome

Nutritionists believe that women who experience severe pre-menstrual syndrome (PMS) have abnormally low levels of certain nutrients, including zinc, iron and the B-complex vitamins. As a wholefood with a comprehensive nutritional profile, blue-green algae has been shown to replenish stores of nutrients, thereby reducing the strain on the body during menstruation.

Radiation sickness

Japan's interest in blue-green algae originally stems from its potential as a powerful detoxifier, which could be used in the treatment of radiation sickness following the atomic bombing of Hiroshima and Nagasaki.

Japanese scientists have shown that blue-green algae is particularly effective in eliminating the heavy metals mercury and cadmium. AFA is an especially powerful detoxifying agent and works well on the liver. Studies have shown that AFA's cellular structure remains stable even at levels of radiation much higher than human cells could withstand. AFA's cells only begin to mutate when exposed to one-hundred times the amount of radiation a human cell could stand.

However, research has shown that after only two generations of reproducing itself in mutated form (blue-green algae can reproduce itself several times in the course of a day), it manages to reverse the process and reproduce normally. Scientists believe that AFA's remarkable life force can not only assist cellular stability in the body and remove traces of heavy metals, but it can also protect the body's cells from the effects of radiation.

Russian doctors treating children suffering from radiation sickness after the Chernobyl nuclear reactor disaster in 1986 have also reported very encouraging results with spirulina. Doctors at the Minsk Institute of Medical Science in Belarus found that 5mg of powdered spirulina taken daily for twenty days helped reduce radioactivity levels in the children's urine by 50 per cent and also reduced levels of lead and mercury (see Chapter 8). As a result of this work, the government of Belarus has awarded spirulina a patent as a medicine for treating radiation sickness.

Senility

Many doctors believe that senility is the result of long-term nutritional deficiencies. Many report that when elderly people are given blue-green algae, they experience improvements in their circulation and increased vitality and energy.

Japanese biochemists, meanwhile, claim that blue-green algae's incredible facility in detoxifying the body, stabilizing cellular metabolism and boosting the thymus gland make it a powerful tool for prolonging human life. Tests have shown that the life-span of mice who take blue-green algae is increased by up to 50 per cent.

This may not be as far-fetched as it seems, as Dr Benjamin Frank, a pioneer in research into ageing, has shown that the loss of energy and physical deterioration associated with ageing are due to the break-down of nucleic material – DNA and RNA – needed to keep cells healthy. Thus a drop in the efficiency of cellular regeneration, caused by toxic overload or poor diet, can affect our life-spans.

Dr Frank found that by putting his patients on a diet of DNA/RNA-rich foods, such as sardines, fish, wheatgerm and green, leafy vegetables, they regained energy, memory and a more youthful appearance. Blue-green algae has significantly more RNA than sardines, one of the highest available sources of RNA, which contain 590mg per 100g.

Ulcers

Blue-green algae contains a chemical called mesafirine, which Japanese scientists claim can inhibit the growth of ulcers. For patients suffering from ulcers, studies indicate that blue-green algae can cure all the symptoms of gastric ulcers and significantly improve the symptoms of patients with duodenal ulcers.

The well-balanced and easily digestible protein, vitamins and minerals in blue-green algae also make it a perfect food for ulcer patients whose diets are restricted because of their condition.

Visual problems

According to Japanese ophthalmic surgeons, around 90 per cent of cataracts in elderly people improved when the patients were treated with a combined programme of blue-green algae and drugs.

Blue-green algae, as we have seen, contains high levels of beta carotene. Recent studies in the US have shown that when high doses of beta carotene are given to people who are extremely light-sensitive (a condition known as erythropoietic protoporphyria or EPP), more than three-quarters of them said they could tolerate light much more easily: some claimed that they could spend four times longer than normal in the sun. This breakthrough was especially important for children who are affected by the disease, as it means they can play outside in the light without becoming sick.

Chapter 5

OUR BODIES, OURSELVES

Health and weight loss using blue-green algae

*Over-eating is like deadly poison to any constitution and is
the principal cause of all disease.*

Moses Maimonides (1135–1204)

As the twelfth-century Jewish healer Moses Maimonides well
understood, the greatest threat to our health after illness and
infections is over-eating. For the developing world, where
grinding poverty and food shortages have left much of the
population close to starvation, this is not the issue. However,
in the West, where food population has accelerated over the
last fifty years, many of the illnesses that are the cause of premature death can find their roots in over-eating and poor
quality food.

As we saw in Chapter 1, world health is in crisis.
Environmental pollution, stressful lifestyles and drugs causing
immune system breakdown have been added to the explosive
cocktail of high-fat, low-nutrient food. Heart disease and
cancer now account for two-thirds of all premature deaths in
the West. Both killer illnesses can be traced back to these significant changes in our diets and lives.

Over-eating can put tremendous strain on all our bodily
systems. The body treats food in much the same way it would
treat a virus or infection – as a foreign body which must be
attacked, broken down and, finally, eliminated. When we

eat, our body must suspend its normal work of repairing tissues and ensuring that all its systems are in balance in order to deal with the food. Once the food has been broken down into its constituent elements, the body can go back to its maintenance work.

However, when we succumb to a serious illness, like a virus, the body automatically overrides the appetite in order to deal with the virus. Thus we do not feel hungry for a few days while the body fights the illness. As soon as it has cleared, we become hungry again.

Unfortunately, too many people pay little attention to their body's need to recover in between eating. Many people will happily eat all day long, without thinking about the traumatic effect it can have on the body. If the body's eliminative and digestive organs are required to work full-time, they never get the chance to rest and renew their cells.

Thus, people who constantly eat large quantities of sugar can find that they develop diabetes in later life because the sugar has caused their pancreas to become stressed. Similarly, people who eat large amounts of fat – as well as possibly developing coronary disease – may find that they suffer irritable bowel syndrome or cancer of the colon or bowel, due to toxic by-products of fats remaining in the bowel for too long before being broken down and eliminated.

At the other extreme of the spectrum are those who eat too little or crash diet in an effort to stay slim and then binge. Scientists are now linking slimmers' diseases such as anorexia nervosa and bulimia in teenage years with the onset of chronic fatigue syndrome and other debilitating conditions in later life. They are alarmed by the growth in advertising which portrays the only acceptable healthy body with an ultra-slim physique – now even men and children as young as six or seven (as well as women) are being conditioned to regard their bodies as imperfect.

Most of us, happily, fall between these two extremes. We may over-indulge at certain times of the year and put on weight through inactivity or during periods of stress. At other times, we may try to pull ourselves up and go on diets in an effort to lose weight quickly. None of these things are good for our health, of course, and in this chapter we shall look at ways blue-green algae can help us improve our general health and encourage the body to return to its natural weight through gentle and controlled weight loss. As it is probably the most perfectly balanced and nutrient-rich food on the planet, blue-green algae is an ideal partner in the fight to maintain health and sustain natural and long-lasting weight loss.

First, though, it is important to get an overview of the way we perceive ourselves, our health and weight. We must realize that society's idea of a perfect shape is not a realistic notion. If we look back over this century alone, we will soon see that shape and styles come in and out of style as quickly and transiently as fashion itself.

A hundred years ago, the idea of dieting for health and beauty was unheard of. For centuries, societies all over the world had gauged each other's prosperity by their weight and stature: the fatter a man was, the richer he probably was. The same applied to women: it was a mark of shame for a man to have a thin, scrawny wife – beauty lay in a generous figure, which had been gently rounded with rich food and expensive wine.

Although many societies still live by these rules, particularly in Africa and the Middle East, definitions of what constitutes a perfect figure is constantly changing in the West. Fashion has been the great catalyst for change, exploding with new ideas and 'looks' during the last seventy years. During the 'roaring Twenties' women abandoned uncomfortable corsets and bodices, which were so tight they often fainted, and had their hair cut into short, manageable styles. But women also had to conform with the new body 'style' as the boyish, flat-chested look became the vogue. For many women, this look was completely unnatural and practically unachievable, but they nevertheless strove to meet fashion demands by wearing tight bands across their chests.

Everything changed again in the 1940s, when a good silhouette in trousers was the height of chic, and the 1950s, when a tiny waist was a woman's most prized asset. In the 1960s, many of the fashion styles of the 1920s reappeared, and what was fashionable in the 1960s is coming back into fashion today in the 1990s, with the revival of the gamine, 'waif' look and boyish fashions.

Although many women claim not to be bothered by fashion trends, it is becoming increasingly difficult to escape them. We are constantly bombarded by images of the 'perfect' female or male physique on TV, in newspapers and in magazines, most of which bear no relation to how most people look. Surveys have found that the majority of women in this country are dissatisfied with their figures, and a growing number of men are unfavourably comparing their less-than-perfect physiques with the images that appear in glossy magazines.

The result of this is that more people than ever – especially women – are going on diets in an effort to improve their figures. Some middle-aged women have been on diets since their teens and have tried every crash diet invented in an effort to lose weight. Although it is teenage girls and young women who seem most preoccupied with diets, men are also beginning to join their ranks, with teenage boys suffering from the dangerous slimmers' diseases anorexia nervosa and bulimia as well as girls. Most alarming of all, however, is the recent trend for children to be concerned about their body shape. Children as young as seven or eight (both boys and girls) are suffering from slimmers' diseases.

Not surprisingly, a whole industry has developed to cater for the so-called 'needs' of dieters: there are hundreds of meal replacements, slimming foods, bulking agents and low-fat breads, sweets and ready-made meals for sale in supermarkets, health-food shops and chemists. Worse, 'miracle' diet aids, such as magic teas or pills guaranteeing weight loss, have cost many gullible – and desperate – people thousands of pounds, with no visible effects. More sinister is the emergence in recent years of slimming drugs that do help people lose weight, but which can have alarming side-effects, such as nausea, headaches and hallucinations, in the long term.

The way to optimum health

Everyone wants to experience optimum health, but how do we do it? The answer can be found in the miraculous cells of our own bodies. All our cells are perfectly equipped to remove wastes and toxins, nourish themselves and regenerate to build new and healthy cells – if we feed them the right quantity, quality and balance of nutrients. When they receive these nutrients in the right balance, the result is good health for the whole body. The more we support our own living cells, the more they will support us. However, when we fail to do our bit, the system can get out of balance, resulting in discomfort, fatigue, irritability, immunological deficiencies and, eventually, disease. Although drugs may alleviate the symptoms of these conditions, they rarely address the root cause of the problem.

David Howell, a homoeopath and director of Aqua-

Source, which distributes blue-green algae in Europe, says: 'Having owned a health-food shop, I have seen so many products that were claimed to be wonderful and ended up not being so.' But there was a sudden improvement in the patients he had been treating homoeopathically when they also started eating blue-green algae. 'I deduced that although I had prescribed the right homoeopathic remedies, their bodies did not have the right nutritional balance to use them. When they started to take blue-green algae, the remedies began to work properly.'

The effects of over-eating

Over-eating in general, especially excess protein and eating late in the evening are two sure-fire ways to blunt the power and energy of the mind and body. The body–mind life-force becomes drained because it has to divert essential energy to support the over-strained digestive system and compensate for low cellular oxygen from blood sludging with fats.

As we saw in Chapter 1, many people in the West have lost sight of what constitutes a healthy diet. As the food industry has become more commercialized, it has become more and more difficult to see beyond advertising campaigns for processed and fashionable foods and choose products which are nutritionally sound. More emphasis is placed on fast, convenience foods, which are rich in fat, salt and sugar, than simple, whole and nutritious foods, such as lean meat, fish, cereals and grains.

The more we eat high-fat foods packed with 'empty' calories, the more depleted our bodies become of the essential vitamins and minerals we need to keep healthy. Under the weight of fatty, non-nutritious food, the body sluggishly searches for nutrients and, when it cannot find them, it triggers cravings for more food. If the body is still fed poor, 'junk' foods, it will rapidly become locked in a vicious cycle of craving food and over-eating in a desperate attempt to find nutrients. Soon, the digestive system becomes clogged, the intestines overloaded with toxins and the weight begins to pile on, raising blood pressure and cholesterol levels and putting the vital organs under stress.

There are some good habits worth adopting. Avoid eating more than the system can easily digest and assimilate and avoid food and drink that disagree with the stomach. Pay attention, too, to the quality and quantity of the foods you eat. Leave the table while still wanting to eat more. Eat when you are hungry and drink when you are thirsty; equally do not eat when you are not hungry and do not drink when you are not thirsty. Allow time for complete digestion between meals – around four to five hours.

The roots of disease

The human body actually treats food in the same way as it would tackle a virus or infection – as a foreign body which has to be contained, destroyed and eliminated. If the body is constantly forced to metabolize food, it will have very little spare capacity to maintain and repair its own systems or fight illnesses. If toxins and waste matter build up more quickly than they can be eliminated, it can soon become a breeding ground for serious illnesses. The reason why fasting can be so beneficial to the body is because it gives the body a chance to rest and rejuvenate itself (see The blue-green fast below).

Many scientists agree that serious degenerative illnesses, including cancer, heart disease, arthritis and multiple sclerosis, either have their roots in poor diet or are more likely to develop when people who are genetically disposed to them eat a diet that is low in essential vitamins and nutrients.

The alkaline/acid ratio

Some nutritionists also believe that many diseases are caused when the body's acid/alkaline ratio is out of balance. Cancer cells, for example, can survive better in a highly acidic and low-oxygen environment than normal cells, and it is thought that cancer is exacerbated when the body's fluids are more acid than alkaline. Acidosis (excess acid in the body) occurs when too many acidic foods are consumed, such as meat, grains, dairy foods, fats, sugars, processed foods, coffee and alcohol. When the body is unable to excrete acid, it stores it in the joints, where it can use up calcium and cause arthritis, and in the muscles, where it absorbs potassium and sodium, leading to severe tension and muscle spasm. As the body becomes more acidic, the nervous system begins to shut down, causing general fatigue and sluggishness. Moreover, excess acid in the blood can cause weakness and lack of mental clarity.

Blue-green algae is one of the most alkaline foods in the world, along with ripe fruits and vegetables. A good intake of these can quickly reverse the symptoms above and prevent long-term damage to the body's systems. One immediate effect is to rid the body of a good deal of stored tension and aches and pains that many people accept as a normal part of daily life.

Scientists suggest that the optimum ratio of alkaline to acid foods should be 80:20, that is, we should eat four times as many alkaline-based foods as acid-based foods. For many people, the exact opposite is true, eating far more acidic than alkaline foods. Consider the average fast-food meal: hamburger (protein/fat) with roll (refined flour) and garnish (acidic tomato ketchup and limp lettuce), chips (high-fat, salt) and soft drink (high acid).

The dangers of crash diets

Existing on a diet of grapefruit and boiled eggs for three weeks may help you get into a particular dress or pair of trousers, but it will not help you in the long term. As well as being unhealthy and unbalanced, rapid weight loss does not have a lasting effect.

Many people who do manage to lose weight on rigorous diets find it almost impossible not to put on the excess weight once they go back to their normal diet. Most find that they pile on even more weight than they lost in the first place. This can breed desperation and result in a yo-yo existence of dieting and bingeing, which can put tremendous stress on the body as well as being very damaging psychologically. Most doctors nowadays advise gradual weight loss, of between one and two pounds each week, by following a carefully balanced diet.

Sudden weight loss with crash diets or diet drugs is very stressful and can have many adverse effects on the body. Research shows that common diet drugs containing phenyl-propanolamine (PPA) may become addictive and can have dangerous side-effects on the kidneys and heart.

New research is also indicating that people who have experienced rapid weight loss may also be at risk where degenerative diseases are concerned. When dieters lose weight very quickly, their bodies release toxins into the system. Unless these toxins are thoroughly eliminated, either by drinking lots of water or through the use of enemas, they can put intolerable strain on the body's systems.

Equally, some researchers are now linking chronic fatigue syndrome and ME (myocardial encephalomyelitis) to the slimming diseases, anorexia nervosa and bulimia, claiming that when the body falls below a sustainable weight, it begins to cannibalize tissues, which may harbour powerful toxins that could poison the system. Moreover, a severely malnourished body does not have the energy to fight both the toxins and opportunistic illnesses that may occur, such as 'flu, viruses or bacterial infection, and the immune system can become permanently impaired.

The psychology of eating

Of course, eating is more than satisfying hunger: meals can be important social occasions and an effective way of bringing people, whether friends or families, closer together. Most people enjoy their meals as a pleasurable, daily event and a chance to indulge themselves in a small way.

However, for some people, eating can become a way to suppress pent-up feelings or emotions. Food can be wonderfully satisfying and, like alcohol, can blunt the edge of painful feelings. Some people eat in an attempt to make them feel better; others may eat in an effort to deaden themselves to the realities of their lives or as a deliberate attempt to self-destruct.

Sweets, chocolate and junk food create the illusion of fullness, contentment and, initially, positive feelings. However, these feelings are usually temporary and, when their effects have worn off, can leave a heightened sense of emptiness and sadness. In an attempt to recreate feelings of satisfaction, the person will crave the foods again and the vicious cycle will recommence.

Many people, as we have seen, find that their lives become controlled by food. This is a very dangerous situation. It is important to keep a proper perspective on food: it is a vital part of our lives, but it is only one of our needs – relaxation, exercise, company, fresh air, time to be quiet are all important, too. A stable emotional and mental environment allows you to think carefully about what you are eating and how it is affecting you. If you are centred and calm before eating and eat in a peaceful environment, paying full attention to the food, your digestive process will be different from eating when you are upset, angry or depressed. Eating in a calm environment greatly benefits digestion.

Guidelines for healthy eating

Before we consider how we can lose weight, it is important to learn how to eat properly. This is one of the most important lessons to learn for health and is not as difficult as it sounds. The key to success is retraining yourself out of lazy habits and learning good, new habits. **Moderation** is the catchword: there is no need to starve ourselves or deprive ourselves of food we like. But, overall, we should make a conscious effort to choose foods our entire body will enjoy, rather than just our tastebuds. In time, our tastebuds will learn to enjoy healthy, wholesome foods and the benefits for our health and well-being – more energy, clear heads, toned muscles, beautiful skin, clear, sparkling eyes, less PMT and headaches, more resistance to colds and minor infections – are incalculable. Once these good habits have been learned, it will be possible to move on to the next stage – losing weight in a controlled, healthy way.

Nutritionists advise people to eat three balanced meals per day. The best time to eat the main meal of the day is **between 10am and 2pm**, when the metabolism is strongest and our body is functioning at its peak. Many traditional medical systems, such as the Indian Ayurvedic system, advocate this practice. Similarly, it is important not to eat late at night (after 9pm), when the metabolism is slowest and digestion weakest. Another point to consider is to think hard whether you are actually hungry or whether you are just thirsty, as the body often confuses these two signals.

When dieting, it is important to eat a **varied diet**: eating the same things all the time can lead to vitamin and mineral deficiencies and can lead to food cravings and addictions. Addictive foods include sugar, starch, breads, chocolate, coffee, tea.

Try to **avoid toxic food** – white, refined flour, white sugar, cakes, biscuits, pastries, soft drinks and junk foods are very hard for the body to process and are virtually nutrient-free. Avoid packaged food with preservatives and limit your consumption of saturated fats, especially red meats – pork, ham, sausages, fried foods, cooking oil, sour cream, cheese. It is not easy to reprogramme yourself to eat a healthy diet, so accept this fact and just do the best you can in the circumstances.

Try to **be aware** of what you are eating. In modern society, we tend to switch off from our food – eating at convenience and speed – running, walking, standing up or watching TV. The more disconnected we become from our food, the more unbalanced become our food choices. It is extremely important to chew each mouthful several times and to try to eat slowly, setting aside time for the meal.

Choose the **freshest and best foods** wherever possible,

especially organic fruit and vegetables, which contain the highest and best complement of minerals. Organic meat and chicken also taste better and have a different fat content as they come from healthier animals. Eat whole grain cereals and breads, pasta and crackers without added sugar or chemicals, live yoghurt, pure butter, naturally fermented cheeses and free-range eggs. Use extra virgin olive oil for cooking/salads.

Try to make sure you eat **50–70 per cent raw food** in your diet. The more stress you are under, the more fresh, raw food you should eat as this has a higher alkaline content and can reduce acid and toxic build-up in the blood.

Avoid food which burdens your digestive tract and circulatory system. These are **danger foods**. Fish, chicken and turkey are better alternatives to red meat or processed foods, which contain salt, sugar, preservatives and chemicals and have fewer nutrients than fresh foods.

- Saturated fats can add unhealthy body weight and also tax the internal vital organs and arteries.
- Sugar, sweeteners and salt can affect your moods adversely and stress your organs.
- Milk and dairy products can cause mucus, bloating and poor digestion.
- Alcohol has little food value. It can stress vital organs and toxify your entire system.
- Caffeine has no food value, but it can stress the nerves and raise blood pressure.
- Soft drinks have little or no food value. Phosphoric acid, found in many soda drinks, can thin the bones by leeching calcium, while the sodium content makes the body retain water.

Make sure that you drink enough liquids, especially **water**, which is a great detoxifier and essential for proper cell function. Try to avoid bottled drinks, including fruit-flavoured mineral waters, as they can contain preservatives and added chemicals. Freshly squeezed (not concentrated) fruit juice, vegetable juice and herbal teas should be drunk regularly to ensure that the body does not become dehydrated.

Planning your meals

It is just as easy to eat good, nutritious meals as it is to eat bad food – the problem lies in making the effort to develop good habits, which means planning meals and thinking carefully about their nutrient content. With practice, it becomes easy and one of the advantages of eating good food is that, after a short time, you will have more energy and brainpower to put into planning your meals.

- **Breakfast** should be carbohydrate-based. Eat seasonal fruit if the morning is warm and sunny, or a grain-based breakfast – muesli, porridge or cereal – if it is not, as this will give you extra energy.
- **Lunch** is the most important meal of the day. It will give stamina and energy for the rest of the day, so eat well. Try to concentrate on proteins for lunch, as too many carbohydrates can make you sluggish and sleepy.

  Lean meat, fish or chicken should be accompanied by green salad – lettuce, rocket, radicchio, parsley, watercress and mustard and cress contain high concentrations of enzymes that promote good digestion – or steamed vegetables. A sandwich made with whole grain bread and tuna, turkey, chicken, egg, prawns, feta, ricotta or cottage cheese is also good.
- **Dinner** should be based on carbohydrates if you

concentrated on protein at lunch. This balances the types of food the body has to deal with and promotes better digestion. It is important not to over-eat at dinner because the body's systems are slowing down at this time and too much food late at night can interrupt sleep and make you feel tired and sluggish the next morning.

The following foods are good choices for dinner: pasta, jacket potatoes, risotto, millet, buckwheat, noodles with pesto or olive oil and vegetable sauce. Accompany with greens and leafy salad.

- **Natural snacks** such as fruit, yoghurt with nuts, seeds, raisins, oatcakes and rice cakes can be eaten throughout the day in preference to sweets and chocolate. Beware dried fruit, however, as this is very high in sugar and calories.

A balanced diet

While you are learning good, new habits, it is important to understand what vitamins and minerals foods provide so you can make a balanced choice in the foods you eat. Below is a rough guide to the main sources of the most important vitamins and minerals. Make sure that each of these vitamins and minerals is included in your weekly diet.

- **Vitamin A:** Organic liver, green and yellow fruit and vegetables, eggs, live yoghurt, butter and sunflower seeds.
- **B-complex:** Whole grains, brown rice, green vegetables, fish, eggs, whey, nuts, bananas.
- **Vitamin C:** Citrus fruits, berries, tropical fruits, green and leafy vegetables, tomatoes, peppers, watercress.
- **Vitamin D:** Sunlight, oily fish, egg yolk, live yoghurt.
- **Vitamin E:** Sesame and sunflower seeds, organic tahini,

extra virgin olive oil, avocadoes, dark green vegetables, soya beans, whole grains.

- **Vitamin F (unsaturated essential fatty acids):** Sunflower and sesame seeds, linseeds, soya beans, walnuts, pecans, almonds, avocadoes, oily fish such as mackerel, sardines, pilchards, wild salmon, herrings, halibut, whitebait.
- **Vitamin K:** Cauliflower, green vegetables, tomatoes, fish.
- **Bioflavonoids:** White and segment part of citrus fruits, apricots, buckwheat, blackberries, cherries, rosehips, cantaloupe melon, papaya.
- **Calcium:** Live natural yoghurt, nuts, sesame seeds, tahini, pumpkin seeds, sunflower seeds, bony fish such as sardines and salmon, carob, most vegetables, seaweeds.
- **Magnesium:** Nuts, seeds, dark green vegetables, apples, figs, lemons, grapefruit, yellow corn, black grapes, raisins, blackberries, avocadoes, lentils, whole grains.
- **Iron:** Egg yolk, apricots, dried fruits, cherries, green leafy vegetables, watercress, parsley, black strap molasses, oatmeal, red wine, strawberries.
- **Zinc:** Pumpkin seeds, eggs, live natural yoghurt, brown rice, rye bread, herrings, fish.
- **Manganese:** Blackberries, blueberries, tropical fruit (especially pineapples), raisins and other dried fruits, avocadoes, olives, watercress, dulse seaweed, nuts, seeds, kidney beans, peas.
- **Selenium:** Asparagus, garlic, onions, fish, tuna, eggs, brown rice, whole grains, tomatoes, broccoli.
- **Chromium:** Organic potatoes with skins, whole grains, nuts, peas, fish and chicken.
- **Boron:** Root vegetables – parsnips, carrots, beetroot.
- **Copper:** Whole grains, nuts, seeds, vegetables, apricots.
- **Iodine:** Kelp and dulse seaweed, garlic, fresh fruit, eggs,

whole grains, live yoghurt, fish.

- **CoQ10:** Fish, especially sardines, eggs, spinach broccoli, alfalfa, organic potatoes with skins, soya beans, brown rice, buckwheat, millet, most beans, nuts and seeds.
- **Potassium:** Fresh and dried fruit, green leafy vegetables, organic potatoes with skins, nuts, sunflower seeds, whole grains, watercress, bananas, mint.
- **Sodium:** All fresh fruit and vegetables.
- **Chlorine:** Kelp, olives, table salt.
- **Phosphorus:** Fish, poultry, whole grains, meat, eggs, nuts, seeds, soya, lecithin, lentils, beans, peas.
- **Sulphur:** Dried beans, fish, eggs, cabbage, onion, garlic.

General rules for dieting

Dieting should only really be considered when you have mastered the basics of healthy eating, as your body should then be in a healthy enough state to cope with weight loss. The rules of dieting are more or less the same as healthy eating, except that you should try to cut down your food intake and limit high-fat foods, such as butter, cheese and eggs. As before, it is important to keep some perspective on dieting. Food is only one factor in your well-being and much of your happiness depends on other things. Emotional problems and stress caused by unsatisfactory jobs and difficult relationships can cause stress and sap vitality, so tackle those problems too.

Again, at mealtimes, eat a balanced diet of **natural foods**, with as many raw foods as possible as these contain far more enzymes and nutrients, which cooking can destroy. It is also important to **exercise daily** to burn off calories and fat deposits. Find an activity you enjoy – aerobics, tennis, jogging, swimming, cycling or brisk walking. Drink plenty of spring **water** as this will help eliminate toxins from the body.

Breathe deeply to **oxygenate the body**. Again, you should attempt to reprogramme your eating habits and lose weight slowly.

One of the most useful tools for the dieter is a **food diary**. Keep it for a week, initially, before you begin your diet, writing down the weight of everything you normally eat or drink. This will help you to understand your eating patterns and help you become aware of what you eat. As well as recording the kinds of food you ate, make a note of the times you ate and how you felt immediately afterwards and, again, two hours later. This is a useful way of seeing how food can affect the mind as well as the body.

The following rules can also make it easier to stick to a diet:

- **Do not skip meals** or starve yourself.
- Plan **regular meals** and snacks throughout the day.
- Set a **realistic weight goal** that is right for your body type.
- Aim to eat the same amount each day: **don't worry if you fail** – you can always start again the next day.
- Examine your **feelings and emotions** when you eat; food should not be a shield for emotional problems.
- Rapid weight loss can result in excessive loss of lean tissue and a reduction in strength, muscle endurance, so **go slow**.
- **Limit your diet** to a month at a time: prolonged dieting or food restriction can lead to menstrual irregularities and amenorrhoea in women, reduced testosterone production in men, increased stress, fractures and bone loss for those who exercise a lot, chronic fatigue and disordered eating.
- Recommended rate of weight loss is **0.5–1kg per week**.
- The key to appetite control and **long-term weight**

management is a high-carbohydrate/low-fat diet.
- **Yo-yo dieting** can lead to a loss of lean tissue and an increased risk of heart disease.

The blue-green diet

If there is anyone who is a good advertisement for a diet using blue-green algae, it is the Japanese philosopher, Toru Matsui, who survived on nothing but spirulina and algae for fifteen years. He lived well into his eighties and apparently experienced no ill-health from living entirely on blue-green algae.

Toru Matsui's diet was a little extreme, perhaps, but it neatly illustrates the fact that blue-green algae is a perfect food in itself. Combined with a low-fat/high-carbohydrate diet based on whole and organic foods and a little exercise, it can help you achieve your target weight with very little effort.

However, because metabolism and biochemistry are different in every individual, weight losses may differ. Track your weight over several weeks. If you want to increase your programme, increase the amount of blue-green algae you take and eat lighter meals or replace one meal each day with a large fruit or vegetable algae drink. It is important, however, to continue to eat at least two nutritious meals each day.

The joy of dieting with blue-green algae – as I have discovered myself – is that **you are never hungry**. Blue-green algae is such a concentrated and perfect food that it satisfies the body's real need for nutrition. Because it contains so many nutrients, blue-green algae can make sticking to a diet much easier, although it is not a substitute in itself for sensible eating patterns. However, it can **bolster willpower** and improve dietary success in two ways: first, it is a highly concentrated source of protein that is quickly absorbed into the body and, second, it contains polysaccharides that raise blood glucose levels. Since hunger is registered in the brain whenever blood glucose or amino acid reserves are low, regardless of the fullness of the stomach, keeping these nutrient levels high can fool the brain into thinking the body is sated.

According to some doctors, blue-green algae readily enters the bloodstream and signals that the body is getting the nutrients it needs. Since the hypothalamus gland that controls the appetite is triggered by falling blood sugar, keeping nutrients saturated in the blood and preventing precipitous falls of blood sugar can keep the appetite on an even keel.

Blue-green algae contains very little starch or sugar. What carbohydrate it does supply, roughly 10–15 per cent, is primarily in the form of rhamnose and glycogen. These two polysaccharides are easily absorbed by human cells with minimum intervention by insulin, thus placing no strain on the pancreas. Hence they provide **speedy energy** without taxing the pancreas or precipitating hypoglycaemia. The lipids found in blue-green algae are commonly known as glycolipids, meaning that they are composed of a sugar portion and a lipid portion. They also function to provide the body with a uniform level of energy, not an up-and-down energy cycle of the kind that results from sugar. From the point of calories, it is also excellent: there are **only 3.9 calories per gram**, compared with 65 per gram of beef. It is also very rich in iron, which is often found to be deficient in women on low-calorie diets.

If the full spectrum of amino acids is present in relatively equal balance, brain chemistry remains stable with no unusual fluctuations towards emotional extremes. But when any one of the amino acids capable of being transformed into a neurotransmitter is present in disproportionate amounts, the competition among them is such that certain chemicals begin to predominate. When this happens, moods can be manipulated. This is the theory behind certain psychotropic drugs which can induce feelings of bliss, euphoria or paranoia.

Spirulina contains comparatively high values of phenylalanine and tyrosine, two of the amino acids that synthesize brain hormones, for instance norepinephrine. However, in addition to the positive effects of norepinephrine, it can also raise blood pressure and create nervous tension. High levels of phenylalanine and tyrosine can **suppress hunger** in some people by inducing biochemical changes in the brain, which may help dieters stick to their diets.

The ultimate convenience food

Because it is a nutritionally **complete food**, blue-green algae does not have to rely on bulking aids, such as carbomethyl-cellulose or psyllum husks which, when taken before a meal, give a feeling of fullness that discourages over-eating. Many slimming products contain these ingredients and, although they are quite harmless and have helped many slimmers, they do not get to the root of the problem – hunger pangs. Many slimmers complain that even after eating products containing these bulking agents, their hunger returns within an hour or two. Algae appears to coat the lining of the stomach wall and helps it to feel both relaxed and satisfied.

Blue-green algae is also remarkably convenient and versatile. It comes in a number of forms: in powder which can be mixed with fruit and vegetable juices for drinks or added to foods; as tablets and capsules which can be taken at any time, and as granules and flakes that can be added to salads or cereals. In recent years, new combination products have appeared in the US, UK and Europe which are specially formulated to raise energy levels, reduce PMT, improve athletic performance and endurance and develop a lighter appetite. Some companies, such as AquaSource, have developed specific diet products, including nutritionally balanced fruit-flavoured drinks which can be taken as meal replacements.

In the US, New Zealand, Australia, Brazil, Mexico, Japan and Taiwan, it is possible to buy a range of foods that contain blue-green algae. These include producing algae-flavoured snack bars, crisps, biscuits, pastas, fruit and vegetable juices and even ice-cream! Although spirulina-enriched bread is on sale in Sweden and blue-green algae pâté in France and Switzerland, Europe takes a much more conservative view on algae, using it more for beauty products, such as body wraps, skin care products, shampoos, toners and tonics.

Clinical research

So far, clinical studies have shown that blue-green algae is a very good nutritional adjunct to conventional diet programmes, which helps to manipulate the metabolism in several useful ways. Much of the research into blue-green algae's effects on weight loss has been carried out in Europe and the US, where it has long been regarded as an aid to dieting rather than as an all-round health food and healing agent.

A study in Germany in 1986 proved that blue-green algae can curb the appetite. Researchers used fifteen human volunteers to test for any appetite-reducing effects and to observe any side-effects. The volunteers were obese outpatients, who were already following a weight-reducing regime. They took spirulina tablets before each meal three times a day for four weeks, followed by placebo tablets for four weeks.

The study found that six tablets (2.8g three times a day

over four weeks) showed a small, but statistically significant, reduction of body weight averaging 1.4kg. There was also a significant drop in serum cholesterol levels and no adverse effects were found. The researchers concluded that it may be possible that weight can be lost faster by eating spirulina.

At the Center for Holistic and Preventive Medicine in Stanton, California, doctors use blue-green algae as part of their diet programmes. Doctors say that the amino acid structure of spirulina may directly influence levels of neurotransmitters in the brain, particularly those that control ambition, mood and appetite. Specifically, it is thought that the high concentration of phenylalanine appears to actually change brain chemistry in favour of the dieter. Normally, the amino acids supplied by protein foods are broken down during digestion and then reassembled by our own metabolic process to form human proteins. Some amino acids, however, are used directly to synthesize brain hormones that affect mood, a sense of well-being, alertness, energy levels and resistance to fatigue – and sensations of hunger.

The blue-green fast

When you fast, good habits gather like friends who want to help.

Djelaleddin Rumi, Sufi poet

It is hard to enjoy balanced health if our bodies are burdened by toxins caused by air pollution, chemical pesticides, or poor diet. It is important for us to be aware that medical drugs, chemicals and environmental toxins don't just go away: they stay in our bodies and can affect our health and well-being for years. Detoxification programmes help us remove these toxins from our bodies, allowing them to expend energy on nourishing and building healthy cells.

Internal detoxification is vital to optimum health. When we don't eliminate waste, toxins can poison us. This occurs when the colon walls become encrusted with faecal matter, which hampers the absorption of vital nutrients. Worse, old accumulated matter in the colon provides a breeding ground for unhealthy bacteria, which can lead to illness.

It is important to get rid of toxins that may have built up in the body over years. Your body cannot nourish and regenerate healthy cells if it is overwhelmed with housekeeping duties trying to keep the body clean. To understand detoxification, think of the car analogy: imagine driving your car without ever changing the oil or air filter and imagine if you run a car on paraffin (poor diet) instead of premium petrol that it was designed to run on. Even if you use the best fuel, the engine will eventually become clogged with harmful dirt and sludge. Just like a car engine, when we fail to remove harmful toxic material our system becomes burdened.

Many people think that 'detoxing' is simply a fad which has become fashionable in recent years. Yet it is one of the oldest methods of healing the body. Great physicians such as Hippocrates, Galen and Paracelsus used it, and it is an important part of many religions, including Islam, and medical systems (Ayurveda, Yoga). It is still common in continental Europe, where hundreds of people attend health farms and spa centres for their annual fast.

Fasting for one day a week is common practice in traditional societies and in many religions. The purpose of going without solid food for three days to a week or longer is to allow the body to cleanse and renew itself. People who benefit from fasting report a feeling of detoxification that makes them feel physically stronger and psychologically clearer.

Recent research has shown that bowel toxins have a tremendous negative impact on mental and physical well-being. Toxins usually come from a process of internal toxaemia, an overgrowth of putrefactive intestinal bacteria in the small and large intestine. These toxins are absorbed into the bloodstream and from there affect our mental and physical functioning. Intestinal toxaemia is predominantly caused by a high protein, low complex carbohydrate diet. Over-eating, eating late at night and constipation can add to the burden on the system.

During a fast, the eliminative systems of the body, the skin, lungs, liver, kidney and bowels become more active. Because the body is not spending energy digesting and eliminating new toxins in the system, it is able to direct all its energy to eliminating old, accumulated waste products. The increased release is usually characterised by foul breath, body odours, dark urine, increased mucus secretion and foul-smelling faeces. Because of the extra energy freed by resting the digestive system, fasting has a normalizing effect on the biochemical and mineral balance in the tissues and acts as a tonic to the nervous system.

The liver is able to detoxify the body to a certain extent, but when high concentrations of toxins are reached, the liver becomes overwhelmed and toxins can saturate the bloodstream. This can also interfere with brain metabolism – schizophrenics have five times more of a certain toxin in their urine than other people. However, when toxins are removed from the system by fasting, general symptoms such as fatigue, nervousness, gastrointestinal problems, headaches, sciatica, low back pain, allergy, ear, eye, nose and throat congestions, and even cardiac irregularitities can be healed. Fasting is not the only cure for illness, but it can ease the symptoms of many disorders. Russian researchers have cured many so-called incurables by a 65 per cent water fast. Fasting is also an excellent way to overcome drug or cigarette dependency.

The degree of toxic overload depends on the individual and the greater the amount of toxins, the more medical supervision is needed. A person on a high-fat, protein and carbohydrate diet will have to detoxify more than someone who has been on a raw food or vegetarian diet. It usually takes five to seven days for the cell memory cravings for certain foods or substances to subside. After the fast, it is usually much easier for the body to get in touch with what it really wants in terms of nutrients.

How toxic are you?

If you don't consider yourself in need of a fast, stop for a minute and think about the following things – and then reconsider!

- Have you ever felt fatigued for no apparent reason?
- Have you ever felt wooden and lifeless?
- Have you ever experienced flashbacks?
- Do you have trouble thinking clearly?
- Do you ever feel light-headed or spaced-out?
- Do you feel irritable without reason or cause?
- Do you have unexplained aches and pains?
- Do you find it difficult to get enthusiastic?
- Do you ever feel anxious but don't know why?
- Do you experience shortness of breath for no reason?

For anyone who has experienced **any** of the above symptoms, it is time they took a fast. Those who recognize three or less symptoms are experiencing low levels of toxic build-up, while four to seven symptoms can signify significant body pollution.

For anyone who has been feeling sick, has been eating a poor diet or who is feeling stressed or fatigued, a fast is a good idea. Low energy, being overweight, indigestion, headaches, allergies, depression, lack of mental clarity, mood swings, susceptibility to colds and 'flu, eating disorders and concentration problems are further signals.

Fast food

Blue-green algae is the ultimate 'real fast food' because it is very easy to digest and provides energy and stamina during a fast. It also provides all the essential nutrients for the body, which means hunger pangs are not so severe. It is also useful for body cleansing programmes because it is a powerful detoxifier.

Dr Christopher Hills, an American doctor who runs fasting programmes using blue-green algae, recommends the use of algae for fasting – a week's fasting using algae and fruit or vegetable juice will detoxify the body and help lose weight in a safe way. He says:

> *As a source of nutrition during fasting or dieting, it is excellent because it helps cleanse the intestinal tract as well as relax the smooth muscle of the bowels. Fasting with spirulina and mixing it with fruit and vegetable juice is the perfect and most natural way to flush out the system with liquids and chlorophyll without denying the body the nutrients for full and effective metabolism.*

Guidelines for fasting

Fasting requires self-discipline and should be done only for limited periods. The cleansing process can sometimes – but not always – stir up certain symptoms: headaches, diarrhoea, pimples, rashes, fatigue, 'flu-like symptoms, nervousness, reduced appetite and frequent urination. Don't be alarmed – these can be positive signals that detoxification is working. For relief, get plenty of rest, drink more fluids and exercise moderately.

If you experience any of these problems, it is best not to stop the fast, but to work through it gently by aiding the eliminative systems with techniques such as foot massage.

Avoiding caffeine, alcohol and foods that are hard to digest such as those with a high fat content can also aid the cleansing process. Use your common sense and consult a doctor if the pain becomes too severe. It does require a little patience, although many people experience positive effects almost immediately – increased alertness, more energy, less bloating and gas and reduced irritability.

It is also important to break the fast very carefully and consciously. During the fast, the digestive system shuts down and must be restarted very carefully. At the end of the fast, the body absorbs everything much more easily so what we put back into our bodies should really be what we need to rebuild a healthy system. It is a very good opportunity to develop a new diet. Common sense should be used: when it is over, light, simple meals should always be eaten, phasing in heavier meals slowly over a period of several days before returning to the normal diet. A ratio of one day of breaking the fast to two to three days of fasting is a good rule of thumb.

AIDS TO FASTING

- Take an **enema** until the bowels are clear at least once a day. Some health clinics recommend as many as three enemas per day.
- **Brush the skin** for five to fifteen minutes twice daily and follow this with a bath and skin scrub to draw more toxins out of the system.
- Get plenty of **sunshine** if possible, and perform deep breathing exercises to help detoxify the skin and lungs.
- Take some gentle **exercise** during the fast to help activate the system and eliminate toxins. Some people recommend up to three hours per day of exercise such as walking or swimming.
- Take short **saunas or steam baths** to encourage perspiration which helps detoxify the system.

LEVELS OF FASTING

Therapeutic fasts lasting from fourteen to twenty-one days are a great boost to the system, but many people find that this is impossible to achieve within the limits of their lifestyles. For many people, a one- or two-day fast over a weekend three times a year is enough to recharge the system.

The degree of fasting also alters depending on whether you are a meat-eater or a vegetarian, as meat-eaters have many more accumulated toxins in their systems than vegetarians.

- **Meat-eaters** should prepare their bodies for fasting by abstaining from meat one week twice a year to start off with, rather than going on a vegetable and fruit fast.
- Those **abstaining from meat** in this way can switch to

fasting three days at a time once a month, or one day per week, or twice per year for seven days, on fruits, vegetables and juices.

- Those on a **dairy/vegetarian diet** can follow the same pattern as above but use only fruit and vegetable juice fasts.
- Those on a **vegetarian diet** or using fasting as a **spiritual practice** can follow a pattern of four ten-day fasts per year, plus either fasting one day per week or three days at one time per month. The fasts can progress from fruit and vegetable juices to wheatgrass to distilled water.

MEDICAL NOTE

Fasting is not for everyone. If you have any sort of serious illness or acute or chronic disease, you should only fast under the supervision of a doctor or qualified health practitioner.

Pregnant women, nursing mothers, children, old people, underweight people and anyone with special dietary or medical problems should consult their doctor before they begin any detoxification programme.

It is also worth remembering that during a fast, our minds and bodies become much slower than usual, so anyone who has to operate heavy machinery or drive cars, buses or other vehicles, should not fast during working hours.

Blue-green algae recipes

Blue-green algae is something of an acquired taste. For those who first sample it, it can be rather shocking because of its lurid blue-green colour and pungent flavour.

This is particularly true of AFA, which also smells, as one friend delicately put it, of rotting fish. This is probably not an unreasonable assumption, as fish tend to live mostly on algae and, when they decompose, no doubt revert to their constituent form! Spirulina is slightly less pungent, smelling of dried spinach and tasting remarkably like puréed green vegetables when taken in powder form.

For this reason, many people prefer to take blue-green algae as tablets, capsules or flakes, but it is worth persevering either with the powder or liquid forms because these have a much more immediate and energizing effect on the body. Rest assured that in time blue-green algae does become more palatable to take and many people begin to enjoy it after a while.

The important thing to remember when taking blue-green algae in its powdered or liquid forms, however, is that it should never be subjected to heat, as this can destroy the active enzymes which make blue-green algae such a valuable and unique supplement.

Algae will keep well if handled properly. Dry powder absorbs moisture from the air if you leave the container open, so keep the bottle tightly sealed after use. You do not need to refrigerate it, but you do need to keep it in a cool, dry and dark place.

Your body will feel the spirulina within minutes because the powder is naturally digestible. Algae drinks once or twice a day provide quick energy and nourishment between meals or in place of a meal. Nor is it possible to take too much algae – but go easy at the beginning as it is a very powerful detoxifier and may cause headaches or spots on the skin.

If you are using algae to balance your diet and help you eat lighter meals, take the drink/capsules/tablets an hour or so before you plan to eat. If there is a certain time in the day when your energy runs low, take some tablets and see how your body feels two hours later.

As blue-green algae is relatively expensive, it is advisable to use it only in cold food and drinks, as heat can destroy some of its vital nutrients. It is best taken in cold fruit or vegetable drinks, sprinkled on food or blended into dips such as hummus or guacamole. For this reason, I have restricted the recipes below to fruit- and vegetable-based drinks, dips, pastes and cold soups, which can be prepared quickly and economically.

Blue-green energy drinks

The quantities of ingredients and blue-green algae given in these recipes are meant only as a guide. It is important to experiment with them to suit your own tastes. For extra zing, the fruit drinks can take spices such as cinnamon, nutmeg, mint, ginger and allspice, while coriander, fennel, saffron, mint, turmeric, basil, oregano, thyme, chilli sauce and freshly ground pepper can be added to the vegetable drinks. Plain yoghurt, soya milk, honey, wheatgerm, desiccated coconut and blended fruit can also be added to the fruit drinks. (All recipes serve one unless otherwise stated.)

Starter shake
1 banana
Half a glass soya milk
Half a glass apple juice
1 teaspoon (5ml) blue-green algae

Mix all ingredients in a blender until they are foamy. Serve immediately.

Blue-green morning booster *(Serves 2–3)*
1 peeled orange
1 peeled nectarine/peach
Glass of pineapple juice
Glass of coconut milk
1 teaspoon (5ml) of blue-green algae

Put fruits in liquidizer with pineapple juice, coconut milk and blue-green algae and blend well. For extra nutrition, add a tablespoon of chopped almonds or sunflower seeds before blending.

All-day energy shake *(Serves 2–3)*
225ml plain bio yoghurt (sheep/goat's milk is best)
Handful of strawberries/raspberries
1 teaspoon (5ml) honey/blackstrap molasses
1 dessertspoon (15ml) coconut milk
Squeeze of lemon juice
1 teaspoon (5ml) of blue-green algae

Combine all ingredients in a food processor. Dilute with apple or pineapple fruit juice if required. Bananas, mango, pineapple, raw egg yolk and natural wheatgerm can all be added for extra energy.

Berry dream
1 apple
5 large strawberries
10 raspberries
10 blackberries
1 teaspoon (5ml) blue-green algae

Juice the apple, pour into a blender, add other fruit and blue-green algae and blend. Serve chilled.

Blue-green pineapple and pears
1 pear
1 apple
1 thick slice of pineapple, chopped
1 teaspoon (5ml) blue-green algae
Sprig of mint

Juice pear and apple and liquidize with pineapple and blue-green algae. Serve chilled with sprig of mint.

Coconut shake
Half a large pineapple
Milk of one coconut
Fresh, grated coconut
1 small banana, mashed
Grated nutmeg
3fl. oz (80ml) soya milk
1 teaspoon (5ml) blue-green algae
Pineapple chunks for garnish

Juice pineapple and add to other ingredients and blend. Serve chilled, garnished with chunks of pineapple.

Kiwi shake
2 small pears
1 kiwi fruit
Half a small mango
1 teaspoon (5ml) blue-green algae
Sprig of mint

Juice pears, kiwi fruit and mango. Blend well with the blue-green algae and serve chilled with chopped mint to garnish.

Savoury shake
8fl. oz (225ml) V8 or tomato juice
1 teaspoon (5ml) blue-green algae
Squeeze of fresh lemon juice
Dash of Worcester or Tabasco sauce
Celery for garnish

Mix all ingredients in a food processor. Serve chilled with garnish of celery.

Blue–green dream
1 stalk celery
6 kale leaves
2 tomatoes
Half avocado, mashed
1 teaspoon (5ml) blue-green algae
Sprig of oregano, chopped

Juice celery, kale and tomatoes and add to other ingredients and blend. Serve with chopped oregano.

Cucumber and avocado cooler
Half small cucumber
Half avocado, chopped
2 fl. oz (50ml) Greek yoghurt
1 teaspoon (5ml) blue-green algae
Fresh mint
1 slice cucumber

Juice cucumber in a juicing machine and add to other ingredients in a blender and blend thoroughly. Serve with mint sprig and cucumber garnish.

Watercress booster
2 tomatoes
Quarter of a large cucumber
Handful of watercress
1 teaspoon (5ml) blue-green algae
Sprig of basil, chopped

Juice the tomatoes, cucumber and watercress. Strain and blend with the blue-green algae and decorate with chopped basil.

Thai zinger
Quarter of a large cucumber
2 large carrots
Half a lime
1 red chilli
1 teaspoon (5ml) blue-green algae
Sprig of coriander

Juice cucumber, carrots, lime and chilli. Blend with blue-green algae and serve chilled, garnished with coriander.

Carrot top
1 tomato
2 sticks celery
2 large carrots
Half a lemon
1 teaspoon (5ml) blue-green algae
Sprig of parsley

Juice tomato, celery, carrots and lemon. Add blue-green algae in blender and serve chilled with a sprig of parsley.

Blue-green salads, dips and soups

Many of these recipes are for dishes made with green foods, such as cucumber, watercress or avocado, so the distinctive colour of blue-green algae does not overpower the dish. As for the drinks, it is best to experiment with the quantities of blue-green algae you add. The quantities given are only rough guides and should be amended to suit your own tastes. As a general rule of thumb, start off with lower amounts of blue-green algae and work up to larger quantities once you have become accustomed to the taste. Either AFA or spirulina can be used, or even a mixture of both.

Tabbouleh *(Serves 4–6)*

2oz (50g) fine burghul (cracked wheat or bulgur)
3 medium-sized ripe tomatoes, finely chopped
¼oz (10g) finely chopped parsley
2oz (60g) finely chopped onions
4 tablespoons (120ml) fresh lemon juice
1.5 teaspoons (7ml) salt
4 tablespoons (120ml) olive oil
1.5 tablespoons (45ml) finely chopped fresh mint
5 teaspoons (25ml) blue-green algae
Cos lettuce leaves to garnish

Place burghul in bowl and cover with cold water. Soak for ten minutes and drain through sieve or colander. Wrap in muslin and squeeze to get rid of excess water. Put the burghul in deep bowl and mix in tomatoes, parsley, onions, lemon juice and salt. Before serving add olive oil, mint and blue-green algae and toss gently until thoroughly mixed. Serve in deep bowl or on cos lettuce leaves.

Iranian yoghurt, vegetable and herb salad *(Serves 4)*
1 medium-sized cucumber
1.5 tablespoons (45ml) finely chopped green pepper
1.5 tablespoons (45ml) chopped spring onions, including green tops
1.5 tablespoons (45ml) chopped fresh tarragon
2.5 teaspoons (12ml) finely chopped fresh dill
Half teaspoon (2ml) freshly squeezed lemon juice
Pinch salt
2 teaspoons (10ml) blue-green algae
2 tablespoons (30ml) plain yoghurt

Peel cucumber and slice lengthways into halves. Scoop out
seeds and discard; chop and place in a deep bowl. Add green
pepper, spring onions, tarragon, dill, lemon juice, salt and
blue-green algae and stir well. Add yoghurt and turn vegetables and herbs with a spoon until they are well coated. Cover
with foil and chill for an hour before serving.

Aubergine dip *(Serves 3–4)*
1 medium-sized aubergine
3 tablespoons (90ml) fresh lemon juice
1.5 tablespoons (75ml) tahini
1 large garlic clove, peeled and finely chopped
1 teaspoon (5ml) salt
2 teaspoons (10ml) blue-green algae
2.5 teaspoons (12ml) olive oil
1oz (30g) finely chopped onions
1 tablespoon (30ml) finely chopped parsley

Prick aubergine in three or four places and hold it on a fork
over a gas flame until the skin begins to char and split, or place
on baking sheet and grill until it chars thoroughly. When the
aubergine is cool, skin it, cutting away charred spots of flesh.

Cut lengthways and chop finely. Blend flesh in liquidizer and add lemon juice, tahini, garlic, salt and blue-green algae. To serve, place in dish and sprinkle with olive oil, chopped onions and parsley.

Tzaziki *(Serves 6 or more)*
1 cucumber, peeled and cubed
1 tablespoon (30ml) salt
1–2 cloves of garlic, peeled
1 heaped tablespoon (35ml) chopped mint or dill
1 teaspoon (5ml) lemon juice or white wine vinegar
3 teaspoons (15ml) blue-green algae
17fl. oz (500ml) natural yoghurt
4 tablespoons (120ml) double cream

Put cucumber in a colander and add salt. Weigh down with a plate and leave for an hour, then drain on paper towels. Crush garlic, with a little salt, until it forms a paste. Add to mint/dill, lemon juice/white wine vinegar and blue-green algae. Stir in the yoghurt and cream. Add cucumber before serving and season to taste.

Guacamole *(Makes 600ml/1 pint)*
4 ripe, firm tomatoes, chopped finely
10 sprigs fresh coriander, chopped finely
Half an onion, chopped finely
2 green chillies, chopped finely
Juice of 1 lime or lemon
1 teaspoon (5ml) salt
Half teaspoon (2ml) black pepper
1 large, ripe avocado
4 teaspoons (20ml) blue-green algae

Mix tomatoes, coriander, onion, chillies, half the lime or lemon juice, salt and pepper. Leave for half an hour. Cut avocado in half and scrape out flesh. Mash with a fork and stir into tomato mixture. Immerse avocado stone in mixture to stop it going brown. Sprinkle blue-green algae over top and fold in lightly. Pour remaining lime or lemon juice over surface and cover. Pour off excess juice before serving and stir. Serve with nachos.

Pesto *(Makes 300ml / ½ pint)*
17fl. oz (500ml) basil leaves
2oz (60g) pine kernels
2 cloves of garlic, sliced
2 teaspoons (10ml) blue-green algae
⅓ pint (180ml) olive oil
1oz (30g) grated pecorino cheese
1oz (30g) grated parmesan cheese
1 tablespoon (30g) butter

Blend basil, pine kernels, garlic, blue-green algae and half the olive oil. Blend into a paste, then add remaining olive oil, cheeses and butter. Stir into pasta or use to season vegetables.

Tapenade *(Makes 300ml / ½ pint)*
4oz (100g) black olives
5 salted, whole anchovies or 10–12 canned anchovy fillets
3 tablespoons (90ml) capers
4 teaspoons (20ml) blue-green algae
8 tablespoons (240ml) olive oil
2 tablespoons (60ml) brandy
1 tablespoon (30ml) lemon juice
Black pepper

Put flesh of stoned olives into blender. Drain canned anchovies or soak whole anchovies for half an hour and remove fillets for use. Add olives and anchovies to blender, with capers and blue-green algae. Blend, adding olive oil slowly and then faster as the mixture thickens. Add brandy, lemon juice and pepper last of all to taste. Serve on toast or bread with hard-boiled eggs.

Gazpacho *(Serves 8)*

1lb 9oz (750g) ripe tomatoes, peeled and chopped roughly
1 cucumber, peeled and roughly chopped
2 green peppers, de-seeded and chopped
1 small chilli pepper, de-seeded and chopped
3 cloves of garlic, crushed
9oz (250g) fresh wholemeal breadcrumbs
5 tablespoons (150ml) wine vinegar
6 tablespoons (180ml) olive oil
4 teaspoons (20ml) salt
1 teaspoon (5ml) chopped sun-dried tomatoes or 1 tablespoon
(30ml) tomato purée
1 tablespoon (30ml) blue-green algae

Mix all ingredients except sun-dried tomatoes/purée and blue-green algae in a bowl with your (clean) hands. Blend in food processor until it reaches your preferred consistency — chunky or smoother. Add sun-dried tomatoes/purée and blue-green algae, up to 750ml of water and seasoning to taste. Chill for at least two hours before serving and add ice-cubes or iced water immediately before serving.

Lettuce soup *(Serves 4–6)*

2oz (50g) butter
9oz (250g) lettuce leaves, shredded

1 medium onion, finely chopped
1 pint (600ml) chicken stock
Salt and pepper
1 teaspoon (5g) sugar
2 teaspoons (10ml) blue-green algae
Bechamel sauce
½ pint (300ml) milk
1 onion
4 cloves
4 peppercorns
Pinch grated nutmeg
1oz (25g) butter
1oz (25g) flour

Melt butter in a saucepan, add lettuce and onion, and cook gently for ten minutes, stirring occasionally. Add stock, and salt and pepper to taste, and sugar. Simmer for thirty minutes in covered saucepan.

Make bechamel sauce by heating milk gently in saucepan and adding the onion stuck with cloves, the peppercorns and nutmeg. Bring to boil, then turn off heat and leave to stand in covered saucepan for fifteen minutes. Strain. Melt butter in small pan and stir in flour. Cook, stirring, for one minute, then remove from heat. Gradually add warm milk mixture, return to heat and bring to boil, stirring constantly.

Add bechamel sauce to lettuce, mixing well, and simmer for ten minutes. Cool, then blend in blender with blue-green algae. Chill for two hours, then season to taste and serve with croutons.

Chapter 6

HIGH OCTANE ENERGY

How blue-green algae can boost exercise regimes

*Those who think they have not time for bodily exercise will
sooner or later have to find time for illness.*
Edward Stanley, Earl of Derby (1826–93)

Most people are now aware of the benefits of exercise, even
if they may not be able to summon up the energy to partici-
pate. Few doubt that there is a direct link between exercise
and good health. Exercise strengthens the immune system,
protects against osteoporosis and brittle bones, improves circulation and flow of oxygen to the cells, balances cholesterol and
blood pressure and can relieve depression and anxiety. It has also
been found to lessen the risk of heart disease, reduce the effects
of ageing and boost energy levels.

These benefits can be significantly improved when combined with a good diet. No matter what sport or exercise
you choose, you can improve your standard and get more
out of the activity by paying close attention to what you eat.
When you exercise, your body must begin to produce
energy very much faster than when it is at rest. The muscles
contract more strenuously, the lungs work harder and the
heart beats faster, to pump blood and oxygen around the
body. All these bodily functions require extra energy, which
is eventually given off by the body in the form of heat,
measured in calories.

Whether you are a top athlete or a housewife or executive struggling to keep fit, a healthy diet will improve performance, endurance and stamina. A deficiency of protein, carbohydrates or any particular nutrient or group of nutrients can hamper your progress, while an optimal nutritional intake can be a great advantage. But what is optimal and how can it be achieved?

Of course, everyone has different nutritional requirements which vary according to size, age, sex, activity and individual body chemistry. However, many sports nutritionists now agree that blue-green algae is one of the best sources of instant energy available to athletes or anyone taking regular, strenuous exercise. This is because it contains certain amino acids and nutrients which actively help the body during and after exercise, together with high levels of easily assimilable proteins, carbohydrates and vitamins.

Nutrients for energy

GLA

Foremost among these special nutrients is gamma linoleic acid (GLA), which stimulates prostaglandins, the body's master hormones, regulating functions of the heart, skin, circulation and muscular structure. Correct prostaglandin levels are vital during exercise as they maintain proper bodily functions during periods of heightened activity.

Ferredoxin

Ferredoxin is also present in blue-green algae, which is very useful for those who exercise because it helps promote rapid elimination of carbon dioxide, which causes the breakdown of saccharides in the muscles during physical activity. Saccharides break down when oxygen is absent in the muscle, creating pyrruvic and lactic acids, the main cause of muscular fatigue. The faster carbon dioxide is removed from muscles, the more chance there is for oxygen to travel to the muscles, which can prevent the breakdown of saccharides. Athletes who take 7–10g blue-green algae per day before exercise have reported less muscular fatigue.

Carbohydrates

Fatigue during exercise can be experienced in many forms – lack of speed, slower reaction times, poorer co-ordination and balance, lack of concentration. Fatigue is often caused because the body uses up its energy stores very rapidly and must call upon reserves of energy to fuel the activity. No matter what type of exercise you take, or how fit you are, your body will use up these reserves – glycogen stores – which are made up of glucose derived from carbohydrates.

This is why it is vitally important to increase your intake of carbohydrates, preferably immediately after exercising as glycogen storage is more efficient immediately after strenuous exercise. As well as blue-green algae shakes (page 144), good sources of carbohydrates include bananas, dried fruit, rice cakes, breakfast cereal, chocolate, bread and starchy vegetables.

The fitter you are, the longer it takes for your glycogen stores to become depleted. Anyone who takes high-intensity aerobic exercise will find that fatigue is the result of a build-up of lactic acid in the muscles and depleted muscular glycogen reserves, while fatigue from low- to moderate-impact exercise will derive from depleted muscle and liver glycogen and low blood glucose.

Blue-green algae is particularly useful for athletes who require vast energy reserves, such as runners, cyclists and joggers, for whom a bulky diet of carbohydrates would be impossible and impractical to maintain. Foods high in complex carbohydrates, particularly high-fibre foods, tend to be very filling, making it difficult to eat enough to satisfy their daily requirements. Blue-green algae supplies high levels of carbohydrates without the bulk of high-fibre foods.

Protein

Blue-green algae is also a very good source of easily assimilable protein, which is vital for regenerating body tissue and maintaining muscles, tendons and haemoglobin levels in the blood. Proteins are made up of smaller units called amino acids. There are twenty amino acids in all, and they can be combined in many different ways to produce hundreds of different proteins, each of which consists of thousands of amino acids linked together.

The body is capable of making twelve non-essential amino acids on its own if it has to, but eight – essential amino acids – cannot be produced and must be supplied by the diet. Blue-green algae contains all the essential amino acids the body needs in a highly assimilable and low-fat form.

Although there is much debate about the importance of protein for athletic performance, scientists now agree that more protein is broken down by the body during exercise and consequently people who exercise regularly need a higher protein intake than those who lead a sedentary life.

The longer you exercise, the more protein is broken down by the body and the greater your needs. Exercise is also thought to be a trigger for activating a particular enzyme in the body which oxidizes certain amino acids. The greater the stimulus to the body, the greater the enzyme activation and protein breakdown.

The problem with a high-protein diet is that it can also contain a significant proportion of fat, as dairy products, red meat and other meat products are high-fat foods. As with carbohydrates, which can be bulky and filling, too much protein can be hard to consume and is bad for general health.

For any athlete or body-builder, blue-green algae is a useful supplement because its high protein content helps build up muscles without fat and, being so low in calories, it helps maintain competitive weight.

Vitamins and minerals

Vitamins and minerals are also vital for maintaining vitality and strength. However, they do not provide energy and must be taken in the right balance to enhance health. Regular and intense exercise increases the body's requirements for the vitamins and minerals involved in metabolism (vitamin B), tissue growth and repair (vitamin A and zinc) and the manufacture of red blood cells (iron).

Many vitamins form the essential parts of enzyme systems which are involved in energy production and exercise performance. Others are involved in the functioning of the immune system, the hormonal system and the nervous system.

Minerals are inorganic elements that have many regulatory and structural roles in the body. Some, such as calcium and phosphorus, form part of the structure of the bones and teeth. Others are involved in controlling the fluid balance in tissues – vitally important for athletes to maintain – and the formation of red blood cells.

Our bodies are unable to make vitamins or minerals, so they must be supplied in our diet. Blue-green algae contains the widest spectrum of vitamins and minerals of any food supplement, in a perfectly balanced form.

Antioxidants

There is growing evidence that athletes and people who exercise regularly produce more free radicals than people who lead a sedentary life. Free radicals are atoms or molecules with an unpaired electron, produced by the body during food metabolism. Normally, they do not present a problem to health, but if the body is exposed to excess cigarette smoke, pollution, exhaust fumes, UV light or stress, they tend to generate more free radicals by snatching electrons from other molecules.

When there is a build-up of free radicals in the body, there is a greater risk of disease. Scientists now believe that free-radical damage is responsible for heart disease, cancer, ageing and muscle stress. Free radicals can also damage cell membranes and genetic material, disrupt red blood cell membranes, oxidize cholesterol in the bloodstream and increase the risk of atherosclerosis and heart disease.

The body has some natural defences against free radicals, however. They are called antioxidants and work as free radical scavengers, donating one of their own electrons to neutralize the free radicals. They include enzymes such as superoxide dismutase, glutathione and peroxidase which have the minerals manganese, selenium and zinc built into their structure. Beta carotene, vitamins C and E, and plant extracts such as carotenoids and bioflavonoids are also extremely effective antioxidants.

Blue-green algae is the world's most concentrated source of beta carotene, containing ten times as much as carrots, previously though to be the main source of beta carotene. It also has vast reserves of natural pigments, vitamins C and E and other carotenoids which are easily absorbed into the blood-stream and can act quickly to prevent free-radical damage.

Nutritionists advise that the best source of antioxidants is in natural foods, such as blue-green algae and raw fruits and vegetables, as they contain a wide array of antioxidants as well as vitamins and minerals, unlike synthetic antioxidant supplements. Each naturally occurring antioxidant appears to have a slightly different effect on the body and to protect against different types of cancer and other degenerative illnesses.

A number of scientific studies have shown that athletes who take extra antioxidants in the form of natural foods experience less muscle cell damage, pain, oedema and tension in their muscles after strenuous exercise compared with those who do not.

Fats

Until recently, it was thought that extra weight, in the form of fat, was advantageous for certain sports such as discus-throwing, judo and wrestling. However, excess fat is now recognized as being unhealthy and athletes in almost every sport now strive to acquire leaner physiques. Yet an adequate supply of dietary fat is crucial for anyone taking part in sport as it maintains a healthy body that can withstand the rigours of strenuous exercise.

Some body fat is vital to our survival. Essential fats form part of the cell membranes, brain tissues, nerve sheaths, bone marrow and the fat surrounding organs such as the heart, liver and kidneys. Here, it provides insulation, protection and cushioning against physical damage.

Women have an additional fat requirement, which is stored mostly in the breasts and around the hips. It is involved in oestrogen production and regulates hormonal balance and menstruation. If stores fall too low, as happens with many women athletes, such as long-distance runners, it can lead to hormonal imbalances and menstrual irregularities.

Fat is also an important energy store, which can be drawn on during any aerobic activity, such as running, walking and swimming. An average person has enough fat for three days and three nights of continuous running, although most people would suffer unbearable fatigue before their fat stores were depleted.

Very low-fat diets, of the type favoured by some sports-people, can lead to deficient intakes of essential fatty acids and fat-soluble vitamins. In the long term, fat and calorie restrictions can result in other nutritional imbalances, depleted glycogen stores, chronic fatigue, loss of lean tissue and reduced performance.

Some essential fatty acids cannot be made in the body and must be supplied by the diet. The body then uses these to make other polyunsaturated fatty acids. Many athletes take blue-green algae to supply fatty acids that are not over-burdened with calories. It has a high proportion of essential fatty acids, including linoleic acid and gamma linoleic acid (GLA), which is found in only a handful of foods.

GLA is a precursor for the body's prostaglandins, the master hormones that control many essential bodily functions, including regulation of blood pressure, synthesis of cholesterol, and the proliferation of cells. All of these functions are, of course, heightened during exercise and need to be monitored with care. Taking a regular supplement of blue-green algae is one way of ensuring that the extra stresses placed on the body by exercise are compensated for with extra essential fatty acids.

Women's special needs

Women athletes and those who take regular exercise need to ensure that they take adequate calcium, iron, vitamin B and folic acid, as even sedentary women can suffer from deficiencies of these vital nutrients. Low body fat levels, amenorrhoea (absence of menstruation) and a low-fat and low-calorie diet can increase the risk of stress fractures and osteoporosis in women.

Women who are involved in sports such as endurance running and gymnastics have a higher rate of amenorrhoea, which is associated with reduced levels of oestrogen, which, in turn, can lead to bone mineral loss. Indeed, scientists have found that female athletes who menstruate irregularly have a lower bone density than women who have normal menstrual cycles. Adequate calcium intake, particularly in the pure form that blue-green algae provides, is thought to offset calcium loss from bones in women athletes.

Iron deficiency is also extremely common among women who exercise. A high proportion of women have low iron stores, which can be exacerbated during strenuous exercise. Iron deficiency can cause fatigue, headaches, light-headedness and breathlessness.

A winning combination

A few years ago, AquaSource, a leading importer and distributor of AFA, conducted a survey on British sportsmen and women who took blue-green algae as part of their diet and training regime. They wanted to see whether athletes could measure any improvement in their performances as a result of taking AFA.

In general, the athletes, who ranged from an army PT instructor to an olympic swimmer and triathlete, found that blue-green algae significantly boosted their energy and endurance levels and eventually improved their performances in competitive sport.

Here are some of the responses, detailing the variety of effects that blue-green algae had on the athletes' physical, mental and emotional lives.

Olympic synchronized swimmer

She had been taking blue-green algae for seven weeks and is training full time at the moment. When she first started taking the algae, she got 'flu-like symptoms for a week; then, in the third week, there was a sudden change and she had a lot more energy, recovering from training sessions a lot more easily, spending less time resting. She was able to put a lot more effort into her training sessions, without feeling much more tired.

By about the third or fourth week her appetite went down a lot and she found that she was eating half as much as before, and had lost around 2 per cent body fat. Also, she needed less sleep as she wasn't getting so tired.

In a recent competition for synchronized swimming, she took the algae in advance, and after ten minutes or so had a real rush of energy. She took extra during the competition and it affected her positively – she wasn't tired at all, to her amazement.

Boxer

He had been taking algae for seven weeks, having started at the beginning of the season. With the detoxification he experienced strange dreams – his sleep was OK, but his dreams were really crystal clear. He sweated profusely and had some slight headaches, but soon noticed the benefits in his running.

Usually, he peaked well and has never taken anything to enhance his performance. If he had to lose weight, he would just take lots of vitamin tablets. After each fight, he would always go down with infections – 'flu, cold sores, and so on, and would be out of training for two weeks and then would have to build himself back up, only to have another fight and then go down again. Multivitamins helped this problem, but since taking blue-green algae, he had not come down with anything.

The blue-green algae definitely helped him build up his fitness. Although he still gets ups and downs in training, there were fewer downs than before. Previously, he would be down for a week and now he only has the odd off-day.

PT *instructor*

During the first week of taking blue-green algae, he was suffering from cold and 'flu symptoms, so was unable to train as usual and didn't really feel the effects of the algae. The second week, after recovering, he progressed into the week feeling well. He maintained his training to his normal standard and when he ran he breathed in a lot of oxygen and had loads of energy. When he did weight training, he felt quite strong. He noticed he was losing body fat at the end of the second week.

By the third week, he started to feel very strong and trained harder than he had in the second week and recovered well between training sessions. In this week, around Thursday, he started to feel tired, and put that down to over-training in the previous three days. He had a high pulse rate and was quite tired, so he eased off on Friday and Saturday and by the Sunday he felt really strong again and was looking forward to training on the Monday.

Again in the fourth week, he started off very strong and this continued throughout the week, which was unusual, because he normally trained very hard at the beginning of the week and by Wednesday or Thursday was usually very tired. That week, he carried right through until Friday, feeling very strong and energized. He could train for longer and more easily aerobically. Normally, he would work for a forty-minute training session but now he was working for fifty or sixty minutes.

On the following Monday, he had a cough and sore throat, but it didn't affect his performance and by Wednesday it had gone. His wife, who had not been taking blue-green algae, had had a chest cold for three weeks, and he was amazed his disappeared after just two days. It was a very good week's training: he was training longer and harder than ever before and was losing body fat – also he had not been getting any of his usual cravings at night for extra food or biscuits, chocolate and junk food.

Week five was very good – he had loads of energy. In the past, after training at high intensity, he had always had headaches afterwards, but since taking blue-green algae he had had none. Through the five weeks, he lost 3.5kg in weight and 2.1kg in body fat. He felt very good, very healthy and very mentally active, and he has also noticed that he was more confident in himself.

Triathlete

For many years, he found it hard to train for his three events without leaving himself exhausted and too tired to do anything else. He tried many different approaches to rectify this, all to no avail.

The first thing he noticed after taking blue-green algae was that his sleep improved and he wasn't so tired after training. It seemed to help his recovery from training and also to keep him cold-free. He was pleased to get back into the rhythm of regular training, and, with the all-important rest, he started to improve to the extent that when he completed an international triathlon (something he hadn't been able to do for three years), he was quicker than in previous years and his recovery was remarkably quick. Next year, he will be doing a full season of triathlons.

Canoeist

He had been taking the blue-green for four weeks. He was out of training with broken ribs for the past couple of weeks, but is now doing light training.

In the first few days of taking the algae, he was waking up at 4.30am and just getting out of bed and wanting to go off training. He was wide awake all the time and, when he did hard training sessions, would finish the session and still want to do more. In the past, he had always felt tired afterwards; with the algae, he felt great. A few upset stomachs and slight headaches were the only ill-effects.

Usually, he has 'flu for most of the time while he is training, but so far he is cold-free.

Army PT instructor

He took blue-green algae over five weeks. He was doubtful when he started; however, during the first couple of weeks, he experienced quite strong detoxification – more bowel movements and headaches than usual. He felt no benefits as far as his training was concerned; in fact, in the first week, he felt more tired – he had been running on overdrive and was bringing himself back to normal.

By the third week, he started to notice drastic changes – he had more energy, recovered faster from exercise, slept better at night and awoke feeling refreshed. He could also train more easily every day.

By the start of the fourth week, after spending a week in Wales, he came home and felt on top of the world. He actually had to cut back his training schedule. He had so much energy that he had to watch what he was doing! He lost 3kg and expected his body fat percentage to change as well.

He felt a lot better for taking blue-green algae – and is looking forward to feeling the results over a long period of time. He is feeling a lot more optimistic about life in general since he has been taking the algae and he has much more mental clarity – he wakes up in the morning and is ready to go. He is quite well-known for having a good appetite, but the algae has reduced the amount of food he eats and he has experienced no consequent lack of energy.

Olympic athlete

For the past twenty-two years, he has been involved in sport at all levels, representing Great Britain in the modern pentathlon and competing in the Moscow Olympics in 1980. In 1985, he developed ME, which brought his competitive career to an end.

In 1994, he was introduced to blue-green algae and, to his amazement, within two weeks he felt more motivated. After a month, he felt he wanted to get fit again. In 1994, he went to the Triathlon World Championships in Mexico and was the third Briton home.

He knows now that his body system was giving up because of a lack of good quality nutrition. Blue-green algae gave him back the quality of life that he had been denied for the previous eight years.

Marathon runner

Since she started taking algae she is convinced it has helped her as a runner. She is able to recover more quickly from a training session or a long run and can train hard without the need for a rest. She knocked a minute off her best time this year on a four-and-a-half mile run.

Chapter 7

SOUL FOOD

Awakening the spirit with blue-green algae

> *Food can no longer be seen as calories or proteins, fat or carbohydrates, or any material form only. Food is a dynamic force which interacts with humans on the physical body level, the mind-emotional level and also the energetic and spiritual level.*
>
> Dr Gabriel Cousens, *Conscious Eating*

Although science and medicine have made quantum leaps this century in understanding how our bodies function, the human brain remains something of a mystery. We know that the brain co-ordinates and controls many bodily activities, including movement, sensory input and a wide range of physiological processes. It also acts as the organ for thought, and different parts of the brain have been identified with specific intellectual functions, such as language-learning or calculation.

However, the brain is also inexorably tied up with the concept of 'mind', an aspect or function of the brain which implies a thinking process that sets us apart from animals, which have a power centre for a brain. Since the sixteenth century, philosophers, such as René Descartes, have been deliberating whether the mind is a function of the brain or whether it is part of something less defined, such as a soul, which is distributed throughout the body and which survives the body after physical death.

These arguments continue today, although the analogies have become somewhat simpler since the emergence of new technology. Dr Peter Fenwick, a consultant neuropsychiatrist at London's Royal Maudsley Hospital, who has carried out pioneering work in near-death experiences, believes the mind/soul–brain relationship can be best understood if it is looked at in terms of the brain being the hardware on which the mind/spirit – as software – runs. They are separate, yet dependent on one another.

Current evolutionary theories do not satisfactorily explain how the human brain evolved to be larger and more sophisticated than that of other primates. The human brain/body ratio is four to five times higher than in primates and, relative to the rest of the body, requires up to ten times as much energy as the brains of other terrestrial mammals.

According to a research paper by S.C. Cunnane and L.S. Harbige, the human brain has evolved into its present size because early man had access to a stable and reliable source of food rich in nutrients over a long period of time, with little competition from other creatures. The researchers believe that these nutrients are difficult to find in the terrestrial food chain, but are readily available in marine-based regions. They conclude that early man must have chosen to live close to water – along rivers, coastlines and near oceans – because the quality of food available was higher.

The diet of early man would have thus consisted of invertebrates, molluscs, small or slow-moving fish – and marine algae. They claim that these foods would have provided man with an abundant source of protein, vitamins, minerals and polyunsaturates, which allowed the brain to evolve to a high level of sophistication and complexity. Other uniquely human features, such as our relative hairlessness, the fact that we walk upright on two feet and that new-born babies have a thick layer of subcutaneous fat also support this theory of aquatic origins.

M.A. Crawford of the Nuffield Laboratory of Comparative Medicine in London believes that animal life evolved in an environment that was rich in fatty acids. He says that the differences between the species were not the result of different chemical reactions, but the extent to which the brain was developed. Around 60 per cent of the human brain and nervous system consists of fatty acids, a statistic which separates us from other animals and which, he believes, accounts for our more sophisticated evolution. As we saw in Chapter 3, blue-green algae contains significant quantities of essential fatty acids, including gamma linoleic acid (GLA). Seeds of plants, such as sunflowers, are another extremely rich source of fatty acids which would have been available to early man.

Interestingly, the first animals to evolve on Earth after algae colonized the planet and produced oxygen by photo-synthesis had a photoreceptor in their brains – a mechanism which allowed them to store and use light. Of course, algae used sunlight to create food from gases such as carbon dioxide and nitrogen which it trapped from the atmosphere and fixed in its tissues. Early marine and terrestrial mammals, it seemed, possessed the same facility, suggesting that light is an important food source.

The importance of sunlight

Nobel Prize Laureate Dr Szent-Gyorgi believes that the life process begins as a little electrical current sent to us by sunshine. Without light, there is no health. US doctor and author Jacob Liberman says in his book *Light: Medicine of the*

Future: 'The medicine of our future is light – we are healing ourselves with that which is our essence.' If we accept this, we can trace a direct evolutionary link back to our most distant ancestors, blue-green algae, from which we evolved and which also required sunlight for its existence. This is the key to the healing power of blue-green algae: it heals us because, on a very basic level, it is us and we are it.

As we saw in Chapter 2, blue-green algae was able to colonize the Earth because it learnt how to harness the energy from the sun through photosynthesis to produce food and release oxygen, thereby creating a suitable atmosphere for more advanced life to evolve. Sunlight is the ultimate source of life on the planet – the basic component from which all life originates. It is not surprising to discover, then, that approximately $3\frac{1}{2}$ billion years after blue-green algae, we, too, are realizing that light is the key to good health.

Light is the least dense form of energy in the universe. It carries the full spectrum of stimulation our bodies need for perfect health. It is absorbed into the body through the eyes and directly through the skin and converted into energy and nutrients. Nerve receptors in our eyes send information contained in sunlight via optic impulses to brain centres – the pineal and pituitary glands and the rest of the endocrine system, which regulates the body's hormones, body cycles and rhythms.

Although most sunlight is absorbed through the eyes, scientists believe that a lot of energy can be absorbed directly through the skin: it is possible that the red blood cells, haemoglobin, in our capillaries at the surface of the skin absorb sunlight directly, just as plants absorb sunlight directly through chlorophyll molecules in their tissues.

Many researchers believe we are bringing sickness upon ourselves because we have managed to disconnect ourselves from natural sources of light, living and working under fluorescent lights, following indoor lifestyles and using glasses, contact lenses, and suntan lotions to protect us from the sun's rays. Some doctors, like Dr Liberman believe that humans in the twentieth century are suffering from mal-illumination, a condition like malnutrition, whereby we are deprived of the nutrients sunshine brings.

Although we are now aware of the dangers of over-expo-sure to sunlight, which can sometimes result in skin cancer, we must also understand that sunlight is important for our health and well-being. The UV rays of sunlight on skin react with ergosterol (a pre-vitamin D substance) to form natural vitamin D in the body. The sun also balances the biorhyth-mic, hormonal cycles of the body and research done on people with cataracts shows that many are the result of hor-monal disorders.

Doctors are also recognizing that sickness and psycho-logical disorders can result from a lack of daylight. Many more people are being diagnosed with seasonal affective dis-order (SAD), a syndrome which causes depression, irritabil-ity, insomnia, fatigue and general listlessness in people during winter months, when the daylight hours are short and they cannot absorb adequate sunlight.

According to Dr Liberman, we need between thirty and sixty minutes exposure to sunlight each day: wearing sun-glasses is not recommended as they block our reception of the full spectrum of sunlight and keep it from entering our eyes.

Full spectrum light is so essential to proper hormonal function that some experts claim that women who were pre-viously unable to become pregnant soon became pregnant when they ceased to wear sunglasses.

Although excessive ultraviolet light can cause health problems, such as skin melanomas, research suggests that completely blocking UV light can actually suppress our immune systems. According to Dr Liberman, UV light increases cardiac output, improves blood profiles of people with atherosclerosis, reduces cholesterol, helps with weight loss and is helpful in treating conditions such as tuberculosis and in destroying infectious bacteria.

Light therapy is used by Germans and Russians to treat lung disease and there are hundreds of studies that prove the health-promoting properties of light. In the *Lancet*, Helen Shaw reports that people working outdoors, even at high altitudes − which increases exposure to the sun − had half the incidence of melanoma that people working indoors experienced with fluorescent light.

High-energy food

Dr Gabriel Cousens, an American doctor and author who has carried out ground-breaking work on diet and health using AFA, believes a vegetarian diet is closer to natural sunlight than processed foods or animal protein and thus balances electrobiomagnetic levels in the body, which in turn restore the balance in cells. He says in his book *Conscious Eating*: 'We are human photocells whose ultimate biological nutrient is sunlight.' A wholefood diet rich in raw foods and live enzymes is a powerful healing force for the body.

Dr Max Bircher-Benner, the Swiss doctor who invented muesli, also concluded that the closer food is to natural sun energy, the higher nutritional benefit it has for humans. He placed plants, which derive most of their food from sunlight, at the top of the nutritional scale and animal food at the bottom, with dairy products coming somewhere in between.

On a more spiritual note, Rudolf Steiner, the Austrian

social scientist and founder of anthroposophy, was convinced that plant nutrition connected humanity to cosmic forces. He believed that nothing could cloud the nervous system when the body was nourished by a vegetarian diet and that plants could take humans out of the mundane world into cosmic and divine realms.

Dr Cousens in *Conscious Eating* takes a slightly more scientific approach, but with more or less the same message:

> *Food, particularly plant food, is a condensation of the sun's energy, as well as more subtle energy from the stars and other sources in the universe . . . Scientists have discovered that the surface of the Earth is constantly bombarded by radiation from different celestial bodies, including the moon, star systems and other sources of radiation in the universe. Plants take these radiations into their energetic systems and ultimately transfer them to humans when they are eaten by humans. From a spiritual perspective, these energies are simply just condensations of the Divine cosmic energy. In the process of eating food, the cosmic, stellar, lunar and other universal energies stored in the food are released . . . We can experience the whole universe in each bite of food.*

AFA and the mind/body connection

According to Dr Cousens, blue-green algae, particularly AFA, has a marked effect on the brain. Algae is probably the most perfectly balanced vegetarian food on Earth and, being the planet's first photosynthesizer and simpler than most plants, is remarkably well placed to transfer its stores of condensed sunshine to us. Having studied the effects of Lake Klamath AFA on hundreds of people since it was first discovered, Dr Cousens believes it has a marked effect on the brain physiology. More specifically, he believes AFA is extremely effective in balancing the left- and right-hand functions in the brain – namely the logical and intuitive.

From our earliest days, society encourages us to develop left-brain skills: logic, calculation, reason and deduction. Educational systems teach us to learn facts rather than develop our own ideas and to become objective rather than subjective. Of course, some remarkably creative people do break out of this rational straitjacket, but for most of us, the world is ruled by left-brain reason. Naturally, this can have a damaging effect on our moods and personalities – how many people are depressed because they have to work in monotonous repetitive jobs which require no creative or intuitive decisions? Only a very few people can express and develop their creative and logical sides – writers, artists, actors, for example. With the exception of a few lucky or talented individuals, many of these people are either barely making a living or are considered eccentric and out of touch with the real world.

We are meant to live as balanced individuals: our logic and reasoning powers are no more important for our survival than intuitive or creative skills. In fact, we are often storing up trouble for ourselves – both mentally and emotionally – if we ignore our intuitive selves. Sometimes, it is only intuition which can successfully decide for us whether a job is worth taking or whether the person we are dating is the one with whom we should spend the rest of our lives.

Dr Cousens thinks that many people who take AFA experience 'an overall increase in mental alertness, mental stamina, short and long-term memory, problem-solving ability, dream recall, enhancement of the visualisation process and a greater sense of centredness and wellbeing' (from

Conscious Eating). He believes that this synchronization of the two hemispheres of the brain helps people move more easily into the alpha state, a tranquil condition we experience in deep relaxation or meditation.

> *The most unique property of AFA, however, is its effects on the mind-brain function. In my work with AFA, I have observed with myself and with clients that it has an extremely high SOEFF* [Subtle Organizing Energy Field – see page 183] *that seems to regenerate mind, body and energy . . . AFA seems to activate the mind-brain function in about 70–80% of those who use it. It has been a blessing for those who do much mental work. It is also excellent for those doing a lot of high-stress work, or students taking exams. It is not a substitute, though, for healthy living and sleep.*
>
> Conscious Eating

The scientific theory

As a doctor, Dr Cousens is able to put AFA's effects into a clear scientific context. He believes that blue–green algae is one of nature's most powerful sources of brain food. It is worth remembering that the Japanese, considered by many to be the most sophisticated and advanced nation in the world, have a diet which relies heavily on fish, which, in turn, feeds mostly on blue–green algae. Fish has long been described as 'brain food' and perhaps the reason for this is the high quality nutrients it contains, largely derived from algae.

Scientists have isolated the chemicals which constitute this brain food – essential neuropeptides, short chains of amino acids that help the brain initiate certain, vital functions. Neuropeptides function either as neurotransmitters or hormones in the human body. AFA is so remarkable, according to Dr Cousens, because its essential neuropeptides appear to be capable of crossing the blood–brain barrier and directly stimulating the brain's own neurotransmitters.

Our own brains are made up of neurons that are individually no more intelligent than algal cells. The brain's intelligence arises from the interconnectedness of its cells. Simple forms of algae also have a remarkable interconnectedness because they are able to share knowledge by transferring tiny strands of DNA called replicons. These travel through air and water just as signals can be sent from one neuron to another and are received by other algal cells integrating with their DNA and subsequently passing down to new generations.

Given that this algal information-sharing is on a global scale and has been active for a million times longer than human civilization has existed, the human mind would probably be unable fully to comprehend the magnitude of algal intelligence.

Darryl Kollman, from Celltech, explains:

Because blue-green algae is a bacteria, when you eat it, the essential bacteria in your intestinal tract have access to all the information contained in the blue-green algae. Furthermore, it is my opinion that the survival information learned routinely by the blue-green algae is information that we need to survive. It would take us a million years to develop genetic information that would allow us to adapt to excess radiation (for example). Blue-green algae can learn to adapt in a few months in nature and when we eat algae, we have access to that information.

Another scientist who is conducting research into the relationship between the brain and light is the German biochemist, Dr Johanna Budwig. Dr Budwig's research has revealed that wholefoods (raw, unprocessed plant foods) are rich in electrons and act as high-powered electron donors, building up solar resonance fields which in turn attract, store and conduct the sun's energy in our bodies. She believes that photons of sunlight stored in food or from sunshine are attracted by this matrix of sun-like electrons or 'biotrons' pulsating in our bodies.

Dr Budwig's theory of biotrons or sun-electrons is still in its early stages, but she believes that the biotron 'guides' the body's Krebs cycle, which helps produce cellular energy. She also thinks that the human brain can absorb sun-electrons directly from the sun, and some theorists now think that as much as a third of the body's energy comes directly from the sun.

It is not a huge logical step to take, then, to believe that energy from sunlight is in a much purer form if it comes from raw fruits and vegetables. Sunlight energy can be almost completely lost if the sun energy/nutrients have to pass through animals before they reach us. However, plants like blue-green algae have a direct link to the sun and harness its pure energy through photosynthesis. When we eat algae, therefore, it releases its stored light directly into us, boosting the body's sun-electron energy levels and boosting the electrical power of every cell.

Dr Cousens claims blue-green algae (especially spirulina), along with flaxseed, is the Earth's most potent source of solar electrons as it has more power to absorb them than any other food. Interestingly, he adds that blue-green algae grown at high altitudes in high-temperature environments contains more beta carotene, other carotenoids and enzyme systems than other algae and, if consumed, enables the body to absorb high levels of solar radiation safely.

The psychic dimension

The link between food and spirituality is a long and clear one. For thousands of years, different cultures have been aware that the types of food we eat have a subtle effect on our consciousness. The Greek historiographer Herodotus reported as far back as the fifth century BC that grain-eating and vegetarian cultures surpassed meat-eating societies in the arts, sciences and in religious development. He believed that meat-eaters were more angry, war-like and sensual. In many ancient cultures – and some modern ones – specific parts of society, such as religious people, ate special foods to increase their spiritual awareness. Thus the ancient Egyptian priesthood had specially prepared food, while Brahmin priests in India prepare their own food and eat separately from the rest of society.

Similarly, many religions have special rules on food, which must be observed if the devotee is to reach full spiritual awareness. Judaism and Islam have a strict code of conduct for preparing food, especially meat, and proscribe certain foods (or the combination of foods at one meal, such as the Kosher rule that meat and milk must not be served together). Any serious devotee of yoga will fast regularly and follow a strictly vegetarian diet in order to progress spiritually.

Of course, observing a strict religious diet is no indication of spiritual development. Without proper action, thought, meditation, wisdom and love, diet has no context. However, a pure diet combined with the right religious observances can be a powerful step towards spiritual transcendence. According to the famous guru Sri Ramana Maharishi, a regulated diet of pure foods, taken in moderate quantities, is the most important rule of conduct for the person who wishes to acquire a pure mind. He taught that pure and healthy foods nourish the body and uplift the spirit: the body is a temple for the spirit, and, with proper care, it can become a clear channel for spiritual energy. When we eat in a healthy, harmonious way, our ability to commune with nature – and the divine – is enhanced. Pure food brings health for the body first, then peace for the mind and, finally, harmony for the spirit.

It seems that what has been known and practised by ancient cultures for thousands of years has been proved scientifically correct in the twentieth century. As noted earlier in his work with sick and disturbed patients, Dr Cousens noticed that AFA supplements appeared to have a marked effect on the human mind/spirit. As well as being responsible for improving creative visualization, balancing moods, counteracting fatigue, and lifting chronic depression, he found that AFA's ability to pass through the blood–brain barrier seemed to boost the body's upper energy centres – or *chakras* – which are connected with psychic and spiritual unfoldment. Dr Cousens noticed that AFA appeared to have a subtle effect on the spiritual *chakras*, largely because it seems to put the mind and body into a deep state of relaxation and composure which then allows spiritual energy to emanate.

By using acupuncture techniques, Dr Cousens and his team discovered that AFA activated the pineal and pituitary glands. These master glands are associated with higher spiritual energies, intuitive powers and psychic abilities. In *Conscious Eating*, he says: 'It is my feeling that the subtle energy from the [AFA] algae gently stimulates these higher centres and is an additional reason for why this algae is so effective in enhancing meditation.'

Looking at things in a spiritual way, Dr Cousens believes

that AFA itself has a powerful aura and energy which we can tap into when we eat it. This he calls the Subtle Organizing Energy Field (SOEFF), a life-force around every living thing which can be altered by positive or negative energy. Dr Cousens believes that the positive and dynamic interaction of human and plant SOEFFs – especially AFA's – is the key to unlocking mental, physical and spiritual energy – also known as *prana* or *chi* – in our lives. Natural food with live enzymes, vitamins and minerals has an independent life-force which can boost the body's own energy.

However, SOEFFs can be disturbed by physical or emotional upset, stress, fatigue or eating food that is low in natural nutrients, according to Dr Cousens. This leads to poor absorption of food, listlessness, poor cell replication and, eventually, disease. If we eat poor, refined food, we must draw on the body's own life-force to absorb it, thereby depleting our own SOEFF. AFA is therefore especially important for people whose energy or life-force is low, as it provides a potent shot of *prana–chi* and does not draw on the body's own failing reserves. This is the natural way to promote health in sick people.

Dream power

Many people who take AFA report that they have powerful dreams and a sensation of healing or clearing at an emotional level as well as greater energy reserves and mental clarity. This may actually be linked to AFA's effects on the brain, which can act as a storehouse for many old thoughts and ideas.

My sister, Janet Corkindale, a medical student at Sydney University in Australia, has an interesting theory for the bizarre nature of dreams. She believes that one of the brain's functions is to act as a huge, multidimensional filing system – or computer – which is constantly sorting information we pick up during the day. This information may be collected actively, for example by reading a newspaper, or subconsciously, or for no reason other than things happened to us when we were in a certain place at a certain time.

During the day this information is put into temporary filing cabinets, clearing our minds of clutter and enabling us to carry on with our main tasks. However, at night, the brain must find a home for all this information and decides which parts of the brain it must be stored in. As information travels down the brain's neural networks, it meets other information crossing in a different direction and sometimes the two can combine to create a spectacularly bizarre or disturbing dream.

Here are some of the dreams people have recorded soon after taking AFA for the first time.

John, 28, *teacher*

He had an alarming dream about finding himself in the room he had lived in during his first year at university. He was vaguely aware that, even though he was in his late twenties, he had come back to repeat his degree because he hadn't worked hard enough first time. His tutor appeared with a very sombre face, telling him he had to try harder. Reddening, panic overcame him, and he tried to get out of the room, but the door was locked and the tutor had left.

John says he was not very happy during his three years at Cambridge. He felt it was a high-pressure environment and found it hard to compete. He spent a lot of time in his room, not working, but avoiding contact with his fellow students, many of whom were no cleverer than he was, but were much more confident and outspoken. He always regretted that he neither performed well academically nor had a great social life and often thought about what he would do differently if he had the opportunity again.

Jane, 35, journalist

In her dream she was knocking on the door of the house belonging to her first boyfriend, whom she'd finished with in her third year at university. She had not seen him for many years and was surprised to have been invited to his house for lunch. He did not open the door, but his wife did, who led her into a room where he was playing with his three small children. He ignored her and looked up and said she'd aged. Jane looked down at her hands and saw that they were wrinkled, like an old woman's. He carried on talking to his children and his wife. Jane instantly felt anger, jealousy, desperation and panic, and fled the house, but he did not even notice. She woke up feeling anxious, but relieved it was just a dream.

Jane was divorced six years ago and has recently split up with her boyfriend, with whom she thought she was going to share her life and start a family. She admits she is very conscious about her age and the biological clock ticking. Ironically, she split up with the boyfriend she met in the dream because he had wanted to marry her and start a family when she was only twenty-two.

Elisabeth, 61, housewife

She had a dream about sitting her maths school certificate, which she took when she was sixteen. She was in the examination room and the exam paper was written in a foreign script – Russian perhaps. She looked around at everyone else, but no one seemed to be worried, so she tried to teach herself Russian in the three hours she had for the exam – hoping for the best. She was amazed at her coolness.

Elisabeth says she passed her school certificate in maths without a problem, and so cannot understand this dream. However, she wonders if it is related to a deep-seated regret about leaving school without staying on for higher qualifications. She has never really stopped to think about whether she should have gone to university, but sometimes thinks she is capable of more academically than she achieved.

David, 57, writer

He dreamt he flew to Mars with his ex-girlfriend. It was quite exciting, but he was disappointed when they got there because the only newsagent on the planet had run out of cigarettes and he needed a smoke. He told his girlfriend they had to go home, but the space shuttle had broken down and they had to stay. He said, never mind, let's see what it's like here. And he took off and flew around, exploring the universe.

David said he woke up feeling 'fantastic' after the dream. He had recently broken up with his girlfriend, who was very interested in spiritual matters, although he was more down-to-earth. He felt this dream perhaps showed him that he should have joined in her interests more – they could actually be rather enjoyable.

Chris, 44, civil servant

He dreamt that he was a small bird sitting all alone on a large, windswept beach. He was painfully aware that no other birds were near. The flock had all flown away, leaving him panicking and wondering what to do. He just sat there thinking. He did not want to look for them and, anyway, sensed they had left years ago. He felt very depressed for a while, but then decided he had to find a new flock, so he cheered up and flew away.

Chris said he felt emotionally drained when he woke up from this dream. It immediately made sense to him, however. He had long been thinking about giving up his job in the civil service and training for a new career. Over the years he had worked so hard that he had lost touch with many friends and felt very lonely, as well as isolated in his job. He had been feeling depressed, but the dream showed him it was time to pick himself up and move on, both in his work and social life.

These are but a few examples of the vivid dreams people have experienced when they first take blue-green algae. Although some may appear alarming, it is worth remembering that most dream analysts believe that vivid dreams are a sure indication of the body clearing itself on an emotional level.

Moreover, lucid dreams can also give a restored sense of direction in life, as the subconscious warns, provokes and gently prompts us into recognizing the importance of our own intuition, which is all too often crushed by the weight of our rational mind as we rush about on our daily round.

Blue-green algae is a useful catalyst for getting back in touch with our intuition, which, when activated and properly consulted, can act as our guiding light in a busy and confusing world.

Chapter 8

THE FUTURE IS BLUE-GREEN

Blue-green algae's role in the next millennium

> *His [man's] appetite will devour the Earth and leave behind*
> *only a desert . . . whatever befalls the Earth befalls the sons*
> *of the Earth. If men spit upon the ground, they spit upon*
> *themselves . . . contaminate your bed one night and you will*
> *suffocate in your own waste.*
> Chief Seattle's address to US president, 1854

Since the beginning of the Industrial Revolution, the Western world seems to have forgotten the importance of living in harmony with nature. In the last fifty years alone, we have caused more damage to the environment than cataclysmic events caused for all the previous generations of Earth. We act as if natural resources are there for us to exploit as we see fit, and treat nature – the land, seas and animals – as something we must ultimately control. Greed and profit have supplanted notions of compassion and humanity.

The result of fifty years' exploitation of the Earth is that we are now facing an environmental crisis of gigantic proportions. As forests are burned down and pollution from industry, car fumes and charcoal burning release more and more carbon dioxide into the air, heat is being trapped within the Earth's atmosphere and causing global warming. This has already resulted in violent climate fluctuations, such as droughts and floods, all over the world. The use of CFC gases (chlorofluorocarbons in aerosol sprays, refrigerators and chemical processes) is also having a devastating effect on the Earth's protective ozone layer, burning holes over various parts of the world through which dangerous UV rays are contributing to global warming and health hazards.

The environmental group Friends of the Earth estimates that 250,000 tonnes of sulphuric acid fall as acid rain in the northern hemisphere each day, poisoning lakes, rivers and seas and destroying forests. The group also claims that every day 372 tonnes of nets are dumped into the sea by commercial trawlers; 1613 acres of land become desert; 10 tonnes of nuclear waste are generated by nuclear power stations, and tonnes and tonnes of topsoil are washed or blown away. Their statistics also show that around 25,000 people die each day either because of lack of water or from drinking polluted water, while one species becomes extinct every five hours because its habitat has been destroyed. According to US Institute for Food and Development Policy, 60 million people starve to death each year, 14.5 million of them children.

With so many millions starving across the world, these statistics are worse than shocking. Food has become a political issue: it is now grown and produced for profit rather than for people. The West has set the world agenda for eating: now, even the undeveloped world is turning its back on traditional, healthy diets to copy the high-protein, meat-centred diets favoured in the developed world.

As well as following the misguided standards set by the West, Third World countries are also copying our agricultural methods in order to produce food for export to the West, bringing in valuable foreign exchange to set against crippling interest payments from loans. Unfortunately, the long-term effect of adopting our agricultural policy is less food produced for the home market and the devastation of natural resources, resulting in famine and starvation in many regions.

The US alone imports 138 million pounds of beef each year from Central America, representing 90 per cent of all the region's beef exports. Environmentalists have calculated that each burger actually consumes 55 square feet of tropical rainforest, which has to be cleared for cattle to graze, together with two pounds of lost topsoil and 625 gallons of water. The vegetation burned during the clearing process releases around 500 pounds of carbon dioxide into the atmosphere. The situation is even worse in Brazil, where 72 per cent of the country's rainforests have been destroyed to provide land for cattle ranches.

Protein derived from meat and dairy products places a great strain on the Earth's limited resources. In her best-selling book, *Diet for a Small Planet*, the author Frances Moore Lapp estimates that meat-eaters need 4000 gallons of water and 3.5 acres of land to produce the meat and dairy products they consume each day.

Again, according to John Robbins in his book, *Diet for a New America*, raising cattle for dairy food accounts for around 85 per cent of the loss in topsoil and in the US takes up almost half the water used. Livestock also produce around twenty times as much manure as humans (causing high levels of methane gas in the atmosphere) and eat five times the amount of grain and soya as the human population. Robbins estimates that the world's livestock eats around twice the number of calories as humans.

However, it is not just the resources we can see and count that are affected by this greed for meat. As we saw in Chapter

1, modern agricultural methods rely heavily on chemical fertilizers, pesticides and herbicides, which can create long-term health problems in the populations that consume the produce. This eventually puts a strain not only on individuals' health and well-being, but also on the health service which has to deal with the explosion of degenerative diseases caused by poor – or over-rich – diets.

Blue-green algae – helping the environment and feeding the world

Most scientists agree that the only way to reverse global warming and save the Earth's natural resources from complete annihilation is to take the five simple, urgent steps immediately:

- Restrict methane and carbon dioxide emissions into the atmosphere, the two gases responsible for global warming.
- Ban CFC gases to stop the depletion of the Earth's ozone layer, which protects against global warming.
- Halt the destruction of rainforests and coral reefs, which causes carbon to be released into the atmosphere in enormous quantities.
- Limit cattle and livestock populations, which exhaust the world's food resources and put a strain on the environment.
- Plant new forests to bind together and build up the Earth's topsoil and release more oxygen into the atmosphere.

Many countries of the undeveloped world, such as Brazil, have been forced to cut down vast tracts of woodland and rainforest for economic reasons. In these countries, millions of people are dependent on the resulting land and cattle farms for their livelihoods. If this land is taken away from them for reforestation projects, they will starve. Yet the loss of vegetation has meant that more and more poisonous gases are remaining in the atmosphere. As we saw in Chapter 2, all green plants and trees remove carbon dioxide from the air, fix carbon from it in their tissues and release oxygen into the atmosphere. Scientists estimate that around 1 tonne per hectare is fixed in agricultural land and around 3.5 tonnes in a tropical rainforest.

Scientists insist that the only way to cut down pollution and global warming is to plant millions more trees. For example, in 1988, the US World Resources Institute recommended that 52 million new trees be planted in Guatemala to offset carbon dioxide emissions over forty years from a single new American coal-burning plant. Yet blue-green algae has been shown to be the most effective plant on the planet at fixing carbon and releasing oxygen.

According to Robert Henrikson, President of Earthrise, a producer of spirulina, and author of *Earth Food, Spirulina*, 1000kg (dry weight) of spirulina consumed 450kg of carbon and releases 1200kg of oxygen into water and subsequently into the atmosphere. 'At Earthrise farms in the California desert, one hectare produces 14 tons per year, fixing 6.3 tons of carbon and releasing 16.8 tons of oxygen' – truly an environmentally sound crop.

Another, more inventive and perhaps more effective, way to cut down global warming is to encourage more algae to grow in our oceans, seas and rivers. As marine scientists point out, water covers two-thirds of the Earth's surface and ocean algae can convert carbon dioxide in the atmosphere into carbon stored in its tissues, which then feed marine life and help build up coral reefs. Algae could therefore have a massive impact on global warming and produce more oxygen than huge reforestation programmes, which can take years to have any effect on the atmosphere.

It was Larry Switzer, a US scientist who founded the Earthrise spirulina company, who suggested as far back as 1976 that the Third World could benefit from intensive algae-farming. Algae had the perfect profile for a crop that could help with serious food shortages in the undeveloped world. In an idealistic, yet visionary, statement, Switzer said:

> It [the crop] had to be more productive than conventional agriculture . . . adaptable to different climates and cultures . . . appropriate ecologically, economically and socially . . . independent of vested interests in world food production and distribution . . . capable of relying on renewable energy and waste or abundant natural resources. It would have to represent a major expansion of the photosynthetic energy base that supports all life on Earth . . . Finally, it would have to radically improve the supply, distribution and consumption of essential protein to millions of pregnant and nursing mothers, infants and children. It is absolutely critical to provide nutrition to the deprived embryos and infants of the world in order to preserve the precious creative genius that is waiting to be released from each fully developed human mind.

Blue-green algae has an important role in providing high quality protein and nutrients without putting a strain on the environment. It is more efficient at converting resources into protein than either cultivated grain crops or farmed cattle. Moreover, algae, especially spirulina, can be cultivated on marginal land which is neither fertile nor good for grazing. It causes no topsoil erosion and the gram per gram of protein produced requires twenty times less land than, for example, soya beans, forty times less than corn and 200 times less than beef.

This is particularly important because over-farmed land across the world is turning into desert at alarming rates. Global warming is also changing the climate in many regions, bringing drought and creating even more arid land – as much as 15 million acres a year according to some estimates. According to the UN Environmental Program (UNEP), '11 billion acres – 35% of the earth's land surface – are threatened by desertification, and, with them, fully one-fifth of humanity.' If this continues, soon, land in many regions of the world will simply not have the capacity to support conventional crops such as wheat, maize or corn. It is not difficult to see that blue-green algae will be an important crop in the future.

Chronic malnutrition is common in tropical and subtropical regions, where many crops fail because of excessive heat and low rainfall. Yet blue-green algae thrives in such conditions and could provide much-needed nutrition for these communities. As well as containing high levels of easily assimilable protein and the full spectrum of vitamins and minerals, it is also very gentle on the body and can be given to people suffering from chronic malnutrition without adverse effects.

In the Sahel region of west Africa, an ambitious project is underway to reclaim the environment and, at the same time, support the local people. The Swiss group, Association Flamant Vert, has planned a green belt along the Senegal/ Niger Rivers which cut through the African countries Senegal, Mali, Niger and Nigeria. Thirty years ago, this region was extremely fertile and supported millions of people. However, in recent years, overgrazing, drought and fuel shortages (predominantly wood) have meant that 75 per cent of its grazing land has become desert and indigenous tribes have been wiped out.

Association Flamant Vert, which won the European Award for Appropriate Technology in 1987 (sponsored by the joint EC/UN Environmental Programme), has suggested the establishment of thousands of integrated algae systems along the rivers which could support fish populations and transform human and animal waste into nutrients which could rebuild topsoil.

Blue-green algae can also be cultivated in specially constructed farms and in brackish or alkaline water which cannot normally be used for agriculture. Commercial spirulina farms in the US, New Zealand and Thailand and natural alkaline lakes in Mexico and Africa can be exploited all year round for a steady source of high quality protein. According to Robert Henrikson, spirulina protein uses one-third of the water consumed in soya production, one-fifth of corn, and one-fiftieth of beef. He adds: 'Because fresh water is one of the scarcest resources worldwide, algae will become more attractive since it does not compete with needs for drinking or agriculture.'

Spirulina, in particular, grows well in salt water and has the potential to turn thousands of miles of unproductive coastline into high-yielding food-producing regions. Marine algae could easily be cultivated along the coasts of west Africa, Peru, Chile, India and the Mediterranean region to feed both humans and animals, including fish. Many of these areas are close to regions where deforestation, desertification, topsoil erosion and drought have threatened millions of people with famine and starvation.

The Manzanar project on the Eritrean coast of Ethiopia is one region where work has already begun to establish marine algae farms. Salt water ponds have been dug on land bordering the Red Sea where algae is cultivated for shrimp which are then fed to tilapia fish to feed the local population.

Blue-green algae can also be used as a natural fertilizer to restore minerals to depleted soil. As we saw in Chapter 2, blue-green algae is particularly effective in fixing nitrogen to boost yields in rice paddies. In India, spirulina is grown in shallow ponds and harvested when the water evaporates and sold to rice farmers. The natural fertilizer is only a third of the cost of chemical fertilizers yet is said to increase rice yield by as much as 22 per cent. The polysaccharides in blue-green algae also help to restore soil fertility and help it retain water. Indeed, algae is so effective a fertilizer that scientists are now looking at ways of developing special strains which are more expert nitrogen-fixers than even the most sophisticated chemical product.

Humanitarian projects

Blue-green algae is a remarkably versatile food for malnourished people and has been offered as part of humanitarian packages to communities all over the world. Its high beta carotene content has helped thousands of people suffering from eye problems caused by lack of vitamin A, while its protein and B-vitamins have improved the diets of countless people.

A tablespoon (30ml) per day has been shown to eliminate iron-deficiency anaemia, the most common mineral deficiency in the world. It is also the most digestible natural protein food, especially important for malnourished people whose intestines can no longer absorb nutrients properly.

Clinical studies have shown that algae is more easily absorbed than any other food in the world and helps rebuild friendly intestinal bacteria.

Children have benefited from humanitarian donations of blue-green algae in the following countries: Mexico (1973); Romania (1984); Togo (1986); China (1987); Zaire (1990); Ukraine and Belarus (1990–4); India (1991–2). Most of the donations have been made by US companies Earthrise and Celltech.

Since 1990, the California-based Earthrise company has donated spirulina powder and tablets to clinics in Belarus and the Ukraine, which have treated children and adults affected by the Chernobyl nuclear reactor disaster of 1986. Many people in the region are still suffering radiation sickness, presenting severely depressed immune systems and cancer.

Children who have been born since the disaster have also been the victims of radiation poisoning, as much of the land and water in the region is still contaminated by the nuclear fallout, making both a conduit for heavy metal poisoning. Many children have suffered radiation damage to their bone marrow, leaving them severely immunodeficient (damaged bone marrow cannot produce normal red or white blood cells). As a result, they are anaemic and suffer terrible allergic reactions, including violent vomiting and skin disorders.

However, doctors at the Minsk Institute of Medical Science in Belarus administered just five grams of spirulina a day for six weeks to these children, and they made dramatic recoveries. Their immune systems improved significantly, with T-cell counts rising and radioactivity counts in urine falling by 50 per cent.

In 1993, a report on the effects of spirulina on radiation sickness stated: 'The use of spirulina decreases the radiation dose load received from food contaminated with radionucleides Caesium-137 and Strontium-90. Spirulina is favourable for normalising the adaptive potential of children's bodies in conditions of long-lived low dose radiation.'

Another report, by the Grodenski State Medical University in January 1994, showed that in a study of twenty-seven children, consumption of five grams of spirulina each day lowered their levels of Immunoglobulin E (which causes allergic reactions in the body) within six weeks, with no side-effects.

The Russian scientists concluded that blue-green algae dramatically strengthens the immune system and protects against disease. Independent studies around the world appear to back this up: when spirulina (or its extracts) is fed to mice, it increases the power of macrophage cells – the body's first line of defence – and helps them communicate with T-cells to co-ordinate the fight against infection. One study found that extracts inhibited cancer by boosting the immune system, the active nutrients being a polysaccharide (complex sugar molecule) unique to spirulina and phycocyanin (the blue-green pigment found only in blue-green algae).

In 1994, a Russian patent was awarded for spirulina as a medicine to reduce allergic reactions caused by radiation sickness and is now an approved treatment for radiation sickness.

Earthrise and Celltech have also donated spirulina to several humanitarian programmes in the developing world which are tackling the problems of malnutrition.

Celltech donated spirulina tablets to twenty-one patients with nutritional deficiencies in a Bucharest municipal clinic. Patients had suffered chronic weight loss, chronic pancreatitis, rheumatoid arthritis, anaemia, diabetes and other symptoms. Most of the patients who took the spirulina reported that their weight increased and their conditions improved significantly.

Spirulina was also prescribed at the Nanjing Children's Hospital as part of a baby food for infants with severe malnutrition. Doctors found that twenty-seven of the thirty children aged two to six recovered in a short period from bad appetites, night sweats, diarrhoea and constipation.

In 1994, Earthrise began a study in Dakar, Senegal, west Africa, involving infants who were suffering from the effects of severe malnutrition. The children made a rapid recovery, showing fewer eye infections, reduced anaemia, improved endocrine system functioning, increased resistance to disease and better absorption of food.

In India, a study of infants and pre-school children in 1991–2 showed that blue-green algae was an effective cure for minor eye disorders, which are common in the region because of lack of high-quality vitamin A. Spirulina was also effective in reversing oral leukoplakia in tobacco chewers in Kerala, India. The complete regression of lesions was observed in 45 per cent of patients as opposed to 14 per cent of people who did not take spirulina.

Meanwhile, in Togo, west Africa, babies in the village of Farende were given spirulina with water at the local village health clinic. They apparently enjoyed the 'green medicine', which helped them make remarkable recoveries from malnutrition. Nurses from the clinic now sell spirulina at local prices to mothers from the surrounding region who bring their children to the clinic for treatment.

Celltech has donated blue-green algae to a Guatemalan project to feed malnourished children called 'Energia Para La Vida' (Energy for Life). Since then, Celltech reports, doctors have noticed greater alertness and longer attention spans from children who had been suffering from malnutrition.

Another project in Guatemala feeds children blue-green algae with two meals a week at several sites across the country. One of the sites is also planning to foster self-sufficiency in the local community by teaching residents improved methods of agriculture and sanitation.

In Nicaragua, where civil war and natural disasters have devastated the economy, making the country one of the poorest countries in the Western hemisphere, Celltech has also provided spirulina as a food supplement. As many as 70 per cent of Nicaraguan children live in poverty, and death from malnutrition, disease and parasites is common. Since 1992, Celltech has supplied more than 3600 children and old people in the town of Naidime with blue-green algae.

According to Celltech, a schoolteacher in Naidime said that after two months of taking blue-green algae the children began to play games – before, they were so malnourished, they simply did not have the energy. Schoolwork also improved dramatically, according to the teacher.

Another field where there is an urgent need for high-quality food supplements is in orphanages in countries of the developing world and war-torn nations around the world. In 1994, Celltech donated shipments of spirulina to a Dominican orphanage after first arranging for the youngsters to receive parasite medication. The orphanage director claimed that soon after, their physical condition greatly improved. He added that many children who had previously experienced learning difficulties were able to advance to the next level of schooling after taking blue-green algae.

Blue-green algae has also been donated by Celltech to the Naomi Bronstein Children's orphanage in Phnom Penh, which has done much work to care for children orphaned by Cambodia's twenty-five-year reign of terror under Pol Pot. The war has left many children orphaned and the population is now almost 70 per cent female. Old people have also been helped at the centre.

Celltech has also donated spirulina to the Chinese ministry of agriculture, animal husbandry and fisheries which, since 1985, has co-ordinated seventeen national research facilities in an urgent attempt to develop spirulina as a new protein source. Programme goals include developing appropriate production techniques, health-food products and medicinal supplements for its citizens and feed for animals and fish. Production on Hainan Island exceeds several million tonnes per year.

Chinese scientists have discovered that spirulina can replace fish powder in hog and chicken feeds, saving money and increasing growth rates. It also increases the survival rates of fish in aquaculture ponds.

Blue-green algae in space

As we saw in Chapter 2, blue-green algae plays an essential part in regulating the Earth's climate and ecosystems. Indeed, it singlehandedly created the life-inducing atmosphere on Earth, allowing ever more complex life-forms to evolve. This is why blue-green algae is the focus of much research at the US National Aeronautics and Space Agency (NASA). It is also currently being investigated for use in space stations and long space journeys by US, Soviet, European and Japanese space agencies.

NASA chiefs are developing a regenerative life support system called CELLS (Controlled Environmental Life Support System), which could be used to produce food and oxygen for astronauts on long space journeys or in manned space stations on planets where oxygen is limited or non-existent. Because space would necessarily be at a premium either in spacecraft or stations, researchers are focusing on micro-algae which could be grown in small tanks.

Early experiments have shown that shrimps and mice can live in a completely sealed environment with a food supply. Blue-green algae would use artificial light to break down the carbon dioxide exhaled by the shrimp and mice and then release enough oxygen through photosynthesis to enable the shrimp and mice to breathe.

Blue-green algae can also recycle human waste products and use them to produce oxygen. This would solve the problem of disposing of waste material during space travel. As the algae grows extremely fast, it could soon turn human waste into purified water and nutritious food for astronauts. The amount of oxygen produced could then support the crew of the spacecraft.

NASA is not the only national space agency that is using algae in space stations. The former Soviet Union has been experimenting for nearly twenty years with several micro-algae for its own Biological Life Support System. Germany is also using spirulina, chlorella and other algae in its Aquarak project. A joint French–Chinese project is also underway to use blue-green algae to regenerate the atmosphere aboard Chinese Long March rockets.

NASA scientists have also indicated that it is aiming to send humans to Mars by 2018. This date would mark the culmination of a series of missions to the red planet, which began in November 1996. NASA has scheduled at least ten missions to Mars, first manned by robots and then, ultimately, humans. These craft will head to Mars and beyond, seeking out new life forms 100 and 150 light years from Earth.

The trigger for the renewed interest in the Mars space programme came in autumn 1996, when NASA sensationally announced that it had discovered evidence for life on Mars.

Researchers at NASA's Ames laboratory discovered microscopic fossils in a Mars meteorite thought to have landed on Earth 13,000 years ago.

Some scientists likened the spiral-shaped remains of organic molecules and carbon compounds found in the meteorite to fossils of blue-green algae that can be seen in some of the oldest rocks on Earth. This has led some to speculate that blue-green algae was actually seeded on the planet by meteorites from Mars, which landed in the primordial soups of chemicals and gases that made up the earliest environment on Earth. Equally, it may have been similar meteorites from Earth that seeded Mars with primitive life-forms such as blue-green algae. Certainly, it is clear that there was a great interchange between the planets at that time.

As NASA scientist Professor Richard Zare neatly put it: 'Who is to say that we are not all Martians or who is to say that Earth put life on Mars?'

Whether blue-green algae will be used in manned space stations in the future remains to be seen. However, one of the spin-offs of NASA's research is the possibility of solar-powered communities using the same principles of regenerative life systems on Earth. These ecological communities would be designed to produce high agricultural yields, while simultaneously restoring the surrounding environment.

Concepts such as closed bio-shelters and city farming will also use algal technology to become viable alternatives to large-scale capital and oil-dependent agriculture. These small-scale farming models will use algae both for food, recycling and regenerating the atmosphere and will work hand in hand with bio-intensive organic gardens and aquaculture.

These are just a few of the planned uses for blue-green algae which are being considered for the future. As we wait for scientists to unlock its full potential for life in the twenty-first century, however, we can sit back and in the meantime reap the benefits of its extraordinary healing powers and feel its calm and balancing effect on our planet's climate and ecosystems.

As we look out into space and wonder what the next millennium holds for us, we should pause for a moment to consider the words of the first astronauts as they circled the Earth thirty years ago. The Earth, they said, was a wondrous sight when they viewed it from space. It was a beautiful, great orb glittering in the darkness with an iridescent blue-green glow. What they did not realize at the time was that it was the simple micro-organism blue-green algae, which has been patiently maintaining the Earth for 3½ billion years, that gives the planet this wondrous glow.

Chapter 9

PERSONAL TESTIMONIES

Thousands of people all over the world have already experienced the remarkable range of health benefits which blue-green algae can bring. In the Prologue to this book, I described my own experiences when I first began to take blue-green algae two years ago: they included relief from chronic muscle tension, improved circulation, greater mental clarity, weight loss and a general increase in my well-being.

As we have seen from earlier chapters, one of blue-green algae's most fascinating attributes is its ability to heal a wide range of illnesses. Some believe that this is because blue-green algae is actually a bacteria, which has an in-built intelligence. In the same way that bacterial infections can use their intelligence to outwit antibiotics designed to kill them, it appears that blue-green algae can use its intelligence to heal whatever part of the body needs attention. As we saw in Chapter 4, blue-green algae's structure (without cell walls) enables it to permeate our own cells and have a direct, immediate effect. Some nutritionists believe it is so intelligent that it can actually read our DNA – or cell blueprints – and from that deduce what is wrong with us, using its unparalleled stock of natural vitamins, minerals, enzymes and carotenoids.

It will be years before scientists will be able to publish definitive research on the benefits of blue-green algae. Clinical trials have already shown that it is a valuable adjunct in the treatment of cancer, radiation sickness, immune disorders, arthritis, heart disease and digestive disorders and extracts of algae have proved their worth as powerful agents in the control of the HIV virus.

However, we do know that blue-green algae is a powerful detoxifier, a highly nutritious source of vitamins, protein and minerals and that it has no serious side-effects, no matter how high the dosage. It is up to each individual to try out blue-green algae for himself or herself – everyone will have a different set of needs and hence a different experience.

Many people are discovering its life-enhancing effects. The naturalist David Bellamy is said to be a keen fan, as is the Israeli psychic and celebrity Uri Geller. He says: 'I started taking spirulina in the early 1970s because I am interested in vitamins and this seemed to be loaded with nutrients. It certainly made me feel more energised – I found I could run around Central Park [in New York] six times instead of my usual four times. I never liked the taste, I admit, but I kept taking it because it had such a positive effect on me. I also think there's a certain mystery attached to it, which I can't explain.'

Robert Davidson, co-founder and director of AquaSource (a UK company which imports AFA from the US) and a qualified homoeopath, believes that blue-green algae's real value is as a cure for the myriad strains and stresses of twentieth-century living. He says:

> *Most people in Britain are suffering from galloping, hidden malnourishment, a problem which stems from over-farming and the use of artificial fertilizers which drain the soil of nutrients. Blue-green algae is our compensation for living in the 20th century. It is not a miracle cure, it is simply highly nutritious.*
>
> *This fact was borne out in my own practice. When I gave*

*people homoeopathic remedies for various disorders, I found
that they were either not recovering or taking a long, long
time to recover. After eating blue-green algae, the remedies
worked really well. I had not anticipated the fact that malnutrition could slow down and interfere with my homoeopathic remedies.*

Although there is still not a huge amount of clinically proven
data about the health benefits of blue-green algae, there is a
great body of anecdotal evidence which bears testimony to its
powers. Below is a collection of honest, real-life testimonies
to the power of blue-green algae. They range from minor ail-
ments to serious, life-threatening illnesses, but they all have
two things in common – an improvement in the conditions
and an enhanced sense of well-being after taking blue-green
algae. I hope these stories encourage and inspire you to try
blue-green algae yourselves.

Testimonies

Accident trauma/pain relief

'I had a serious car accident in 1987 which resulted in acute
pain in the neck, head and back which lasted until recently,
when I started taking algae. I was taking distalgesics or
coproximol, which, as most people will know, are quite nasty
painkillers – as many as eight in a day. I took the algae in
February and by the next day the pain had receded to such an
extent that I did not need to take any painkillers and since
then, I can count the number of times I have had to take them
on the fingers of one hand. It's only when I have done something really strenuous or made an awkward movement that I
have had a slight twinge. So that is one benefit.

'I have also noticed in the last three months that my sight seems to be improving. I have not been able to read small print from the age of about six – I have had to wear glasses. Now I am able to read small print and books at night without using my glasses, which is something I can only put down to the algae.'

Ageing

'I have been taking blue-green algae – mainly as a vitamin supplement – for the last five years. As well as feeling really well, the remarkable thing is that I don't feel as though I have aged in the last five years. I am fifty now and yet people say I look closer to forty – I don't have any grey hair and the lines on my face don't seem to be getting any deeper. I am not a vain man – and certainly did not start taking algae for this reason – but it's a great bonus.'

Allergies

'I have suffered from hayfever since I was a small girl. I always dreaded summer because I would go around with a streaming nose and puffy eyes for months. I did take antihistamine drugs, but I was always worried about the long-term effects they might be having on my health.

'I am always looking through women's magazines for alternative remedies and I noticed an article on blue-green algae in an American magazine when I was there on holiday last year. I got hold of some and took it avidly. I must say that the effect was not immediate, but this summer I have not been as badly affected by hayfever as in other years. I think it is a gradual thing – your body builds up a resistance over however many years you take it.'

Anaemia

'I suffer from very heavy periods, which leave me feeling weak, depressed and tired for several days of the month. One month last year, my period lasted for eleven days and I had to go to the doctor for medicine to stop it – I was really worried. My doctor diagnosed me as anaemic and, since then, I have followed all his recommendations to boost my iron levels – taking vitamin supplements and eating an iron-rich diet, but that did not really improve things sufficiently. I even tried herbal medicine and acupuncture, but I still suffered painful periods each month.

'Then a friend of mine told me that she had read somewhere that blue-green algae was good for helping with painful periods, so I got hold of some. The first period after I started taking it was still very heavy, but it was not so painful as before. After about three months, I noticed that it was getting easier and easier and that I did not feel as tired, before or afterwards. I am really glad that I discovered it because it has really helped with my anaemia.'

Appetite

'I have been on the algae for a month now and I notice that my appetite has changed quite dramatically. I eat a lot less and I seem to get a lot more energy from what I eat.'

Arthritis / endometriosis / candida

'A friend introduced me to blue-green algae. On days one and two, I only took one capsule, but on days three and four I took two capsules. I didn't notice anything different until day four, and then I realized how it had been working on me.

It's so subtle, I could hardly detect the differences in me, but by day four, this is what was happening:

- My arthritic condition in my back, knees, neck and shoulders which was before a fairly constant aching I had had for seven years was almost indetectable – I felt comfortable and easy.
- I had endometriosis for three years, which I experienced as a pelvic inflammation: a very dense uterus (numb, almost), weariness and, again, aching and irritability. All the symptoms clearly dispersed significantly, to the point where I felt more rested and had a flowing sense of release and relief.
- I had candida which had been recurring for two years and at the time I couldn't seem to change this, no matter what remedies or approaches I tried. By day four, the symptoms of vaginal soreness and itchiness had gone completely.
- All my life – as long as I could remember – I felt the victim of my adrenal glands – I would speed around in top gear too much. I did not feel able to change this at all, no matter how much I relaxed. But after four days of taking the algae, I felt calm and contented, yet very alert and motivated.

I now feel happiness, strength, extra energy, mental clarity and I feel tuned up, tuned in and alive.'

Cellulite

'Although I was very fit as a teenager, I stopped exercising regularly when I went to university and started to put on weight. I have always been able to lose the pounds easily by going on diets, but now that I am in my early thirties, I have developed quite heavy patches of cellulite on my legs and hips which is impossible to shift, no matter how much I diet. I have tried every cream and body lotion available (and have spent hundreds of pounds in the process), but nothing worked.

'I started taking blue–green algae five months ago because I was feeling a bit run down. I noticed that it stopped my food cravings – especially for chocolate and sweet things – and I started to eat less. I was surprised – and delighted – to discover that, after a few months, my legs looked much smoother and firmer. I could not believe that the cellulite was disappearing, but it was, in front of my eyes. I kept checking my legs by pinching the fat, but it really was disappearing. Now I am really pleased with my figure – I look better than I did ten years ago!'

Chemotherapy recovery

'As a cancer patient with four operations and a year's chemotherapy behind me, I would expect to feel very tired for quite a long time, months or even a year – and, to begin with, I did. However, since taking the algae, the tiredness has gone. I feel full of energy and everyone remarks on it. I started taking two capsules a day and now I take four each day.'

Circulation/energy levels

'I am an ex-schoolteacher in my fifties and I took early retirement, thinking that life would just peter down to a slow rhythm, but, with the algae, there has been quite a change. I took two capsules and I noticed that after about twenty minutes, my energy was steadily rising and then settled out.

'More than that, I noticed that my circulation was affected. I was tingling right down to my feet. I also noticed that it had a very calming effect and I was quite nonplussed by that – my energy was rising yet I was calming down. The algae seems to balance the body.

'The day I took the capsules, I had a very severe PMT headache that I simply could not budge. That had started at two in the morning and approximately thirty minutes after taking the algae it had gone. At 9.30pm that evening I still felt alert and wide awake. I didn't know what was causing me to feel so wide awake and it suddenly occurred to me that I was also watching television, but getting none of the eyestrain that I normally experience. My eye muscles were strengthening. My arthritic pain was also diminishing.'

Constipation

'I used to have terrible constipation and have had it for most of my life – I am thirty-seven – but since taking the algae, I have not had it once.'

Depression

'I heard about the algae around three years ago. My stubborn nature stopped me from taking it. I missed out. Now I have been taking it for three months and I am depression-free. My energy is great and my attitude to life is very positive. I use algae to clear low energy levels and headaches and I find that it helps with my digestion. My head now gets fuzzy without it.'

Eczema

'My four-year-old son, Tom, suffers from really bad eczema on his face and it upsets me to see him scratching it and in obvious pain. I had tried everything – from creams to lotions boiled from Chinese herbs – but nothing seemed to work in the long term.

'I came across blue-green algae a few months ago and read in a book that it can help heal wounds if applied externally. Apparently, it was used during the war on soldiers with open shrapnel wounds. I thought I'd give it a try with Tom, so I mixed it with water and made it into a facepack. To be honest, I was staggered, because the eczema seemed to clear up within a matter of days. But the really funny thing was that our dog, Sukie, a Yorkshire terrier, used to lick some of it off Tom's face when I wasn't in the room. I thought it was just a bit of fun (even if it was rather unhygienic!) but she obviously knew what she was doing, as her coat, which had been rather thin and mangy, improved as well!'

Emotional balance

'I began taking blue-green algae two months ago and, since taking it, I have noticed an increase in my energy and personal balance. I experienced some toxic clear-outs – headaches and loose bowels for a short while. I also found it cleared my emotions.

'That has now passed and I am now able to cope with the strain of getting up six or seven times during the night to help my disabled stepson.'

Energy increase/weight loss

'I have been on algae now for two months and have noticed that I have much more energy. I sleep a lot better – I suffer from insomnia, so it has been a great help.

'I also put my children on the algae and they both seem

to have more energy. My daughter is getting better grades at school and my son is a happier person to live with. My husband is also a lot better – he has lost a lot of weight (half a stone), his bad back has improved and he looks a lot fitter. I have also lost three-quarters of a stone. I have my two horses, two dogs and two ducks on the algae, too, and they are all doing pretty well.'

Fatigue/addictions

'I used to suffer terrible fatigue in the morning. I found it very hard to get up and felt tired for about two hours before I could get myself going.

'When I started taking blue-green algae, I began to get up much earlier and now I feel much more energized throughout the day. I have also noticed that I have upgraded my food choices: I had known for some time that it was better to eat fresh fruit and vegetables and healthy foods, but now my body is naturally drawn to eating raw foods.

'I have also become more conscious of my intake of toxic substances – alcohol, nicotine and recreational drugs. I had been trying to withdraw from them for many years, but I found that the algae really helped me to stop. I was just not attracted to using or abusing these substances as much as I used to. In fact, the whole process of getting off some of my addictions has been assisted. I also noticed increased mental alertness, and I think it has helped me emotionally.'

Food sensitivity/sleep

'I have only been eating blue-green algae for about three weeks. I am sensitive to certain kinds of foods, such as mushrooms, red wines or sauces made with brandy or whisky. I need to be very clear in my thinking at work and I often find that I am not because of what I eat – my joints and muscles ache and this affects my emotions significantly. I can be very intolerant can fly off the handle very easily. I have not had these problems recently. If the algae is responsible for that, it is quite extraordinary, because nothing has ever helped me with this save avoiding these kinds of foods completely. It's a great start.

'In exercise or workouts, I also find that I want to carry on for significantly longer periods. Although I sleep well, I am sleeping better and falling asleep more quickly. I am also waking up feeling much more refreshed. I am giving algae to my dog and cat now and they also seem much more energetic.'

General health improvements

'I am an old-age pensioner and about four months ago I was introduced to algae. I have never looked back. I take it every day and so does my wife. She has been quite sick, both mentally and physically, and has felt tremendously better since taking the algae.

'I have also introduced it to a woman who has MS and psoriasis and she is also much better. I can recommend it to anyone. The algae has definitely helped my skin and my general health – I just feel better in every way, more able to cope with everyday life.'

Gum disease

'Two years ago, I was experiencing an unusually stressful time in my life . . . I developed a gum disease which seemed to resist conventional treatment as recommended by my dentist . . . I decided to add blue-green algae to my diet . . . I found myself experiencing more energy and a subtle form of emotional balance which I hadn't expected as the gum disease disappeared.

'When I returned to my dentist for a check-up, she was extremely intrigued to find that not only were my gums clear of infection, but they had become pink and healthy . . . she asked if I could supply her with some algae.'

Hair loss

'I noticed last year that my hair was getting thinner and more and more was falling out when I washed it. Baldness doesn't run in my family − as far as I am aware − and I was worried in case there was something seriously wrong. My doctor thought I was run-down and stressed; he suggested I took some vitamin supplements and I found blue-green algae in the health-food shop. I don't know why I chose it out from the others − I think I was just attracted by the fact that it was completely natural.

'After a week or so, I noticed that my hair was no longer clogging up the shower or sink, nor did it seem to be getting thinner. After a month, I also felt much more energetic, yet calm, and my hair was shiny and − dare I say it − thicker!'

High energy/weight loss

'I started eating blue-green algae three years ago. I began at the deep end, by taking four capsules a day. Within a week, I had noticed some changes happening in my body. I felt less tired, I had more energy and my mood was up. I continued with the same dosage and, over the next few weeks, I observed that not only did those benefits continue, but that I also began to lose my cravings for sugar. I lost a kilo in weight!

'The algae is really powerful – I wouldn't be surprised if my body doesn't start to change at cellular level and possibly even completely regenerate. Time will tell.'

Insomnia

'I am a sixteen-year-old student and have just taken my GCSEs this summer. I go to a very academic school and was under a lot of pressure from my parents to do well in my exams. Just before they began, I got so wound up that I could not eat, sleep at night or even think straight. I was really worried, because I could not get on with my revision and the weeks were rolling on.

'My mum's friend told us about blue-green algae and gave me some tablets. I took them and after a few hours felt quite full, as if I didn't want to eat anything else. That night I managed to get about six hours' sleep – which was a great improvement on the previous night! After a few days, I was sleeping normally, which helped me to get on with my revision during the day. I did really well in my exams, by the way!'

Intestinal disorders/low blood sugar

'I am physically in much better condition since taking the algae – I had bad intestinal problems and low blood sugar. Since taking the algae, all I want to eat is healthy food instead of lots of sweets and chocolates. Emotionally, I had gone through a traumatic time four years ago with a nervous breakdown. When I started taking the algae, it put me in touch with my depression and the breakdown and initially I went through a minor crisis. It helped me to see where I needed to change and I am now going in a much more positive direction.'

Irritable bowel syndrome

'I am thirty years old and last year began to suffer from irritable bowel syndrome, which I had always considered to be an old person's illness. My doctor told me it can also be brought on by stress as the nervous and digestive systems are very closely linked – when one is under stress, the other is affected. That made sense: last year I got divorced, moved house and my father had a heart attack – all in the space of three months. I also work very long hours and live alone. A friend told me about blue-green algae and at first I took it just to please her. After a few days, though, I found that I could sleep better and that I felt calmer. After a couple of weeks, I felt less stressed and began to enjoy my food more. Although I was also careful not to eat too many rich, fatty foods, I felt it was the algae that cured me of irritable bowel syndrome by restoring the balance in my body.'

ME (myocardial encephalomyelitis)

'I started eating algae two years ago. I had had ME for about six years and over that period of time I had tried many different things to try to get well. I had changed my diet, tried many different supplements, Chinese herbs, acupuncture, massage, spiritual healing. I am a qualified hypnotherapist.

'I often felt better for a week or two after the treatment, but then I would be back at square one again. Nothing else seemed to get to the core of the problem. I was going around with a body that felt as if it was that of a seventy- or eighty-year-old woman – I felt like I was driving myself around all the time. I had a lot of difficulty concentrating at times; I live in central London and, some days, just crossing the road was a real effort. I would think: 'I am going to get run over, I just can't focus.' I had headaches a lot of the time and I ached all over.

'When I started taking the algae, the improvement was very gradual. I felt slightly better after about six weeks and I was not sure it was the algae at that stage because with ME you do go up and down. Then, after about three months, I knew it was the algae – I was beginning to feel a lot better, but it took about eighteen months to rebuild my body and it has literally transformed my life. I feel a totally different person.'

'I started eating algae three weeks ago – within three days I noticed a great difference in my health. I have suffered from ME for six years now and my life has been totally destroyed by it. But now I can see a light at the end of the tunnel and it looks quite exciting.

'Three weeks ago, I was an absolute disaster – I was really stressed out – yet now I have committed myself to buying a house even before my other one is sold. My husband asked me for a divorce yesterday, but, even with all this happening, I feel quite happy in myself.'

Memory improvement

'This may sound really strange, but I think my memory has improved since I started taking blue-green algae. Since I was at school, I have been making mental lists about what to do each day – I actually prided myself on not having to write things down. But this summer, I found myself forgetting to do things and got into a real spin. It was a very busy time at work, and I think I was under severe stress. I am also much older – thirty-eight!

'My wife gave me some algae and, although I didn't want

to take it because it tasted terrible, she made me carry on. I did so, just to please her, but after a week I found that my memory was improving and things began to clear in my mind. Now I also write things down when I'm stressed, but I can still memorize a lot!'

Mental clarity

'The main thing I noticed about taking the algae was a real shift in mental clarity. I am in a business where being sharp is really important, so it was wonderful that the algae helped my clarity of thought.'

Migraine

'I have suffered from migraines since I was a teenager (I am now thirty-five). Sometimes they were so bad that I vomited and had to stay in a darkened room for hours until they passed. I tried to watch my diet, but nothing seemed to help except prescription drugs. In desperation one day, I took blue-green algae and found that the pain began to recede almost immediately. I have been taking it regularly for the last six months and I now find that my migraine attacks are less frequent — and far less severe.'

Parkinson's disease

'I started taking algae about eight months ago and my energy levels overall have been considerably higher. I am able to do a lot more with my time and do not need so much sleep as before.

'My mother has Parkinson's disease, which she has had for about seventeen years, and she looks distinctly better since taking the algae. Her eyes have dried up so that she can now read.'

'My father has Parkinson's disease and has been finding it difficult to walk without the help of a zimmer frame over the past nine months. Since taking algae he is walking much more steadily and hardly ever uses the frame to support him. He is looking better and is no longer constipated.'

Pre-menstrual syndrome (PMS)

'I have been taking algae for a month. One of the noticeable things that has happened to me is that I have had no period pain for the first time in my life, with no need for painkillers. I have been more relaxed at night and have also enjoyed eating my food more. I don't get a lull in the afternoon after eating meals and generally feel I have much more energy.'

'I have been taking algae for about three months and I have found that I don't suffer from PMS any more. I don't get food cravings now – they have disappeared. I have also found that I have much more energy at my step class and sleep far better.'

Rheumatoid arthritis/sleep

'I have been eating algae for about eight months. The first thing I noticed after two or three weeks was that I seemed to be sleeping very well – I wasn't having any difficulty falling asleep at night or getting up in the morning. This was very unusual for me. I was also feeling very energetic.

'It was then quite a while after that that the residual symptoms I had had from rheumatoid arthritis seemed to have disappeared. Up until I started taking the algae, whenever I had any incidental illness or if the weather was very damp or wet, my joints got a little bit inflamed or swollen and that is something that hasn't happened to me at all during the last eight months.'

'I began taking blue-green algae in the spring of last year, after seven years of orthodox treatment failed to help my rheumatoid arthritis, which I have suffered from the age of twenty-seven. After taking the blue-green algae, my blood no longer tested positive for the rheumatoid factor. I had a feeling the condition was improving naturally, but the algae certainly accelerated the improvement.

'After my own experience, I gave some blue-green algae to a fellow-sufferer whose condition had been deteriorating chronically for twenty-five years. After a few weeks, she improved dramatically. I am a doctor and I regard her recovery as unprecedented, almost miraculous.'

Scalp problems

'I started to include blue-green algae in my diet three months ago. Within a week, the irritation of my scalp almost disappeared . . . the area round my nose became less greasy and over the weeks, I found that my energy levels increased.'

Skin improvement

'I have been taking algae for about two months and I have more energy than I know what to do with. My skin has become much better – it was rather dry before – and I think I feel much better all round.'

Stress

'I have been taking algae for three months to cope with stress levels at work. I fly a lot and have a fear of flying and the algae seems to combat those fears. It has also made my hair grow and improved my skin and nails. I think it is a wonderful source of food.'

'I dreamed a year ago about a lake and thought that I had to actually go to this lake and even move there. I have friends who have been taking algae for a long time and they recommended it to me about a month ago. Since then, I have moved house and spent three hours running up and down stairs with boxes – I couldn't have done that without the algae. There has been the usual attendant stress associated with moving and getting finances sorted out, but the algae has helped to level me. It has given me strength, stamina and vitality and is evening out my physical self.

'I am very susceptible to colds and 'flu and last autumn I got chicken pox for the first time as an adult, which was horrible. I felt my system did not recover properly from this until I took blue-green algae.'

Surgical recovery

'My mother had surgery for the removal of a tumour in the colon. She had been taking algae for three weeks beforehand and the doctors were absolutely amazed that her bowel knitted back together in just one week and she was functioning normally. Her energy levels are higher than I ever remember and she has a much brighter outlook on life since taking the algae.'

Tinnitus/pain relief

'I began taking the algae three weeks ago. I have had tinnitus for two years and this has now completely cleared up. During the week, I chipped a large piece off my tooth and the nerve is exposed, but I have had no toothache or trouble whatso-ever. Up until recently, my gums would bleed whenever I cleaned my teeth and that has now stopped.

'I was macrobiotic about twenty-five years ago, and I have always wanted to get back to that diet, when I felt really healthy and clear in my thinking. Now I can see that my hands, my skin, everything, seem to be changing. I do eat a wholefood diet, so I am amazed that in just a few days there have been such signs of improvement. I have three children at home, but I feel much calmer than before. Something is definitely happening.'

Weight loss

'I am an alternative health practitioner and I recommend algae to my patients. I have a client who has been on it for three weeks. She has severe arthritis of the knees and is very overweight and depressed – her husband died ten years ago and she has never got over his death. After two weeks, she rang me to say she had been playing music again and feeling much happier. She is also walking better, her knees are not so painful and she is losing weight.

'I also have three cancer patients, two of whom have been told their cancers are incurable. One lady has only been taking it for a week and she has ridden her horses for the first time since she was diagnosed.

'As for myself, my mother died six months ago and I have been very depressed. In the month since I have been taking the algae, I have felt a lot fitter and have lost over half a stone in weight. My husband and daughter are also taking it and they seem much happier. My nineteen-year-old son doesn't like his job, but he has seemed much happier since taking blue-green algae.'

Select bibliography

Barry, Dr WT, *The Astonishing, Magnificent, Delightful Algae,* 1992

Bean, A, The Complete Guide to Sports Nutrition, A&C Black, 1996

Carmichael, WW, "The Toxins of Cyanobacteria", *Scientific American,* January 1994

Challem, JJ, *Spirulina,* Keats Publishing (US) 1981

Cousens, Dr G, *Conscious Eating,* Essene Vision Books (US) 1992; *Spiritual Nutrition,* Cassandra Press (US) 1986

Duff, K, *The Alchemy of Illness,* Virago Press, 1994

Ford, BJ, *BSE: The Facts,* Corgi Books, 1996

Gustafson, K, et al. "AIDS-Antiviral sulfolipids from cyanobacteria (blue-green algae)". *Journal of the National Cancer Institute,* August 1989

Hanssen, M, *Spirulina:* Ronore Enterprises Inc (US), 1989

Hills, Dr C, *Rejuvenating The Body Through Fasting with Spirulina Plankton,* University of the Trees Press (US), 1979

Jassby, A, "Spirulina: A model for microalgae as human food", Cambridge University Press, 1988

Kavaler, L, *Green Magic: Algae Rediscovered,* Thomas Cromwell (US), 1983

Kay, R A, "Microalagae as Food and Supplement", *Critical Reviews in Food Science and Nutrition,* 1991

Kozlenko, R, and Heuson, RH, "Latest Research on Spirulina: Effects on the AIDS Virus, Cancer and Immune System", Dana-Farber Cancer Institute/Harvard Medical School, Boston, 1996

Lappe, FM, *Diet for a Small Planet,* Ballantine Books (US), 1982

Lovelock, JE, *Gaia, A New Look at Life on Earth,* Oxford University Press, 1979; *The Ages of Gaia,* Oxford University Press, 1988

Marsden, K, *All Day Energy,* Bantam Books, 1995

Nakaya, N et al, "Cholesterol-lowering effect of spirulina". Tokai University (Japan), *Nutritional Reports International,* June 1988

Schwartz, J, Scklar, G, Suda, D, "Growth, inhibition and destruction of oral cancer cells by extracts of spirulina". *Cancer and Nutrition,* June 1988.

Switzer, L, *Spirulina, The Whole Food Revolution,* Bantam Books, 1982

Tokai, Y et al, "Effects of spirulina on caecum content in rats". *Chiba Hygiene College Bulletin* (Japan), February 1987

WHERE TO BUY BLUE-GREEN ALGAE

Both spirulina and Lake Klamath Algae (AFA) are available in most good
health food shops. However, it can also be purchased direct from the supplier
in specialist forms, including concentrated liquids, crystals and flakes.
Combined products are also available, such as meal replacements for dieters
(see below). Here are some useful addresses and telephone numbers. Most
products are available by post.

All Seasons
19-21 Victoria Road North, Southsea, Hampshire PO5 1PL
Tel/fax: 01705 755660
Importer of Earthrise green superfoods, mainly spirulina-based products,
including:
Spirulina and chlorella
Spirulina gold (high concentrate spirulina)
Nutragreens (spirulina, chlorella, cereal grasses, flower pollen and lactobacillus)
Barley and wheat grass
Chlorella (green algae)

AquaSource
Carlton House, 27a Carlton Drive, Upper Richmond Road,
London SW15 2BS
Tel: 0181 246 4100   Fax: 0181 246 4101
email@aquasource.co.uk
Produces and imports its own-brand Klamath Lake Algae, most notably
'Lighten Up', its range of meal replacement formulas for dieters, and a com-
parable range for athletes and body-builders. Although some products are
available in the shops, many are sold through direct marketing.
Also available:
Digestive enzymes and algae
Acidophilus and algae
Bifidus complex and algae
Super antioxidant and algae
CoQ10 plus chromium and algae
Protein shakes

Biotech Health
Southview Rectory Road, Great Haseley, Oxford OX44 7JO
Tel: 01844 279100
Spirulina powder, tablets and capsules

Celltech
1300 Main Street, Klamath Falls
OR 97601, USA
American company producing a range of products incorporating AFA. These products are sold through direct marketing. Its range includes:
Liquid Algae
Bifidus-algae capsules
Acidophilus-algae capsules
Combined bifidus/acidophilus algae capsules
Enzymes and blue-green algae
Organic wheat sprouts/AFA/Dunaliena sea water red algae
Blue-green algae and coenzyme Q10
Blue-green algae animal food
Blue-green algae-based skin and hair products

Hunter Ridgeley
26 Churchfields, London E18 2QZ
Tel: 0181 504 7889
Fax: 0181 491 0750
emailbluegreen@usa.net
Flash-frozen and freeze-dried freshwater AFA, imported from US

Institute for Optimum Nutrition
Blades Court, Deodar Road
Putney, London SW15
Tel: 0181 877 9993
     0181 877 9980
Fax: 0181 870 8995
General advice by qualified nutritionalists and specialist clinics

Nature's Gold
783a Fulham Road, London SW6 5HD
Tel: 0171 736 1600   Fax: 0171 384 1759
Lake Klamath AFA, including a highly concentrated liquid form, and combination products, such as:
Acidophilus and algae
Bifidus and algae

Digestive enzymes and algae
High energy protein shakes for children, sick and elderly

Nutricentre (Hale Clinic)
7 Park Crescent, London W1N 3HE
Tel: 0171 436 5122
    0171 631 0156
Fax: 0171 436 5171
A wide range of blue-green algae products, available by post. Credit card orders accepted and same-day dispatch. Open Monday to Friday, 9am to 7pm.

Photosynthesis UK Ltd
The Green Gem Centre, Barrel Sykes
Langcliffe Road, Settle
North Yorkshire BD24 9JT
Tel: 01729 825415
Fax: 01729 825405
Specialist importer of Taiwanese Chlorella, the green algae, a top health food in Japan

Solgar Vitamins Ltd
Chiltern Commerce Centre, Asheridge Road
Chesham, Buckinghamshire HP5 2PY
Tel: 01494 791691
Fax: 01442 890366
Produces several products incorporating spirulina, including:
Earthsource, Greens & More (includes organic grasses, sea algae, Hawaiian spirulina and Chinese Chlorella)
Organic grasses/sea algae (includes dulse, chlorella and spirulina)

INDEX

Goldberg, S.L., 104-5
greenhouse effect, 48
gum disease, 104-5, 215-6

haemoglobin, 84, 86, 87, 98, 173
hair loss, 85, 216
Hale Clinic, 13
Harbige, L.S., 171
hayfever, 208-9
heart disease, 1, 17, 26, 42, 65, 105,
    113, 120, 160, 206
heavy metal pollution/poisoning, 32,
    36, 76, 106, 110
Henrikson, Robert, 192, 195
hepatitis, 108
Herodotus, 181
Hills, Dr Christopher, 139
Hippocrates, 44, 93, 136
histidine, 75, 79
HIV virus, 22, 95-6, 104, 206
Hoffer, Dr Abraham, 85
Howell, David, 118
humanitarian projects, 196-201
hypertension, 65, 101, 106
hypoglycaemia (low blood sugar), 34,
    88, 132

immune system/disorders, 22, 36, 37,
    42, 99, 101, 102, 106-7, 113, 122,
    159, 197, 198, 205
impotence, 42
industrial pollution, 32, 33, 188
inositol, 85
iodine, 129
iron, 19, 33, 39, 49, 62, 66, 81, 86,
    97, 98, 109, 128, 132, 159, 163,
    196
insomnia, 214, 217
intestinal disorders, 217-18
irritable bowel syndrome, 114, 218
isoleucine, 75, 77
Islam, 136
Israelites, 53

Japanese, 19, 53, 56, 58-9, 64, 66, 67,
    68, 69, 86, 94, 95, 98, 101, 103,
    106, 109-10, 111, 112, 134, 178

Kanembu people, 57, 58, 108-9
kelp, 56-7
Khong Minh Khong, 57
Kollman, Darryl, 71, 179

lactobaccilus, 103-4
Lake Klamath AFA, 21, 63, 70-1, 90,
    91-2, 177
Lapp, Frances Moore, 190
LDL (low density lipoprotein), 105
Leonard, Jean, 58
leucine, 75, 77
leukaemia, 31
Liberman, Jacob, 172-3, 174, 175
lipids, 39, 62, 63, 87-8, 132
liver disease, 108
Lovelock, James, 50, 51
lupus, 31
lysine, 75, 77

magnesium, 31, 38, 81, 86, 98, 128
Maimonides, Moses, 113
malnutrition, 52, 94, 97, 108-9, 194,
    196, 199, 200
manganese, 81, 128, 160
Manzanar project, Ethiopia, 195-6
Marathon runner, 169
Mars space programme, 202-3
Matsui, Toru, 131
Mayans, 56
ME (myocardial encephalomyelitis), 5,
    31, 93, 122, 218-19
meals, 124, 140; best time for main,
    124; planning, 126-7
meditation, 10, 15
memory improvement, 219-20
mental clarity, 220
mercury, 32, 110
methionine, 75, 78
Mexico, 54-6, 62, 64, 67, 68, 69, 94,
    197
Microcystis aeruginosa, 91
middle age/elderly people, 66
migraine, 220-1
minerals, 19, 20, 27, 30, 34, 38-40,
    42, 43, 44, 48, 49, 51, 60, 62, 63,